GET WELL,
STAY WELL

GET WELL, STAY WELL

How to beat persistent congestion and infection for good

DR PAUL SHERWOOD

WITH CLAIRE HAGGARD

Thorsons

While the author of this work has made every effort to ensure that the information contained in this book is as accurate and up to date as possible at the time of publication, medical and pharmaceutical knowledge is constantly changing and the application of it to particular circumstances depends on many factors. Therefore it is recommended that readers always consult a qualified medical specialist for individual advice. This book should not be used as an alternative to seeking specialist medical advice, which should be sought before any action is taken. The author and publishers cannot be held responsible for any errors and omissions that may be found in the text, or any actions that may be taken by a reader as a result of any reliance on the information contained in the text, which is taken entirely at the reader's own risk.

Thorsons
An Imprint of HarperCollins*Publishers*
77–85 Fulham Palace Road,
Hammersmith, London W6 8JB

The Thorsons website address is: www.thorsons.com

Published by Thorsons 2001

10 9 8 7 6 5 4 3 2 1

Text illustrations by Peter Cox Associates

A catalogue record for this book
is available from the British Library

ISBN 0 00 710395 6

Printed and bound in Great Britain by
Martins the Printers Ltd, Berwick upon Tweed

CONTENTS

Acknowledgements   vii

Preface   ix

PART I

GETTING WELL, STAYING WELL   1

1   Your Body's First Line of Defence   3

2   A Guide to the Lymphatic System   10

3   Breakdown and Repair   23

4   Helping Your Body to Help Itself: Exercise, Fresh Air and
    A Healthy Diet   30

PART II

A CLOSER LOOK AT LYMPHATIC STRUCTURES AND NODES   59

5   The Tonsils, Adenoids and Appendix   61

6   The Cervical Nodes   82

7   Inguinal, Abdominal and Thoracic Lymph Nodes   93

8   Lifestyle and Lymphatic Overload: Asthma and Its Treatment   101

PART III

A–Z DIRECTORY: PROBLEMS ASSOCIATED BY LYMPHATIC

MALFUNCTION   119

PART IV

LYMPHATIC DRAINAGE TREATMENTS   207

Glossary   226

Index   233

TO ALL MY FAMILY, WITH LOVE

Jane, Robin and Julian Sherwood and
Amanda and Clive Kitson, and
my two grandchildren, Emily and Juliett

ACKNOWLEDGEMENTS

I would like to thank Caroline Trevelyin Johnson for insisting I produce this book and who continued to chivvy throughout the time of its production. Also for her many suggestions as to how the book would be best produced and for introducing me to Thorsons and, best of all, to Claire Haggard.

I especially thank Claire for taking on my complex and random thoughts and turning them into a coherent and artistic whole.

I am most grateful to Tom Donohue for all that he has done in suggestions and moral support and for bringing about a climate which justified the production of the book.

I would like to thank my sons Robin and Julian for the support and encouragement and the many suggestions they have made to the improvement of the book. My wife deserves the reader's sympathy for having her holidays and weekends ruined while I worked to put down my thoughts concerning the book.

And most of all to my Editor Wanda Whiteley for taking the book on in the first place and for nursing it through to its beautiful final state.

PREFACE

I have often been asked how I can claim to be a specialist both in the treatment of bad backs and of recurrent colds and ear trouble. Is it really possible to be expert in two such different medical areas?

The answer is that my approach to the treatment of a particular complaint is quite different from the one generally adopted in the world of conventional medicine today. The tendency in the medical profession is for a doctor to become a specialist in a certain part of the body, such as the eyes or the feet, the abdomen or the chest. As an expert in this field, he or she knows every sort of illness that affects that particular part of the body. Given the bad habit that diseases have of not sticking within strict anatomical boundaries, it makes far more sense, to my mind, to deal with a particular *process* of disease and then look at whichever parts and functions of the body are affected.

The lymphatic system and the sympathetic nervous system – the body's two main defence and repair systems – are the focus of my practice. These two systems are, generally speaking, very efficient at maintaining our health. However, for various reasons – many of which are to do with our 'civilized' way of life, which has created conditions so different from those the body was designed to live in – these systems break down, with repercussions for our health and well-being. The aim of my treatment is to restore the normal function of defective defence and repair mechanisms, so helping the body to do its own job. This is the link between the two areas of my practice and explains why I treat such a broad range of ailments and conditions, from back problems and arthritis to asthma and ear problems.

My patients come from all over the world – a reflection perhaps of the universal lack of understanding of the lymphatic system and the part it plays in various diseases. When I explain the function of the system and how disrupting its smooth running causes particular ailments, my patients feel a sense of relief as they gain a new insight into the working of their bodies.

Often these patients have been told that little or nothing can be done to help them, or that they will have to take drugs to relieve their symptoms – in some cases, for the rest of their lives. By using safe, 'physical' medicine to restore the ailing lymph system, including simple massage techniques which can be carried out at home, I have nearly always been able to help them to enjoy a fit and healthy life free from pain and reliance on drugs. More importantly, equipped with this knowledge they have been able to play a major part in their own – or their children's – recovery.

It is this knowledge and insight that I hope to pass on in this book. Lymphatic problems often arise early in life, which is why this book is aimed particularly at parents. Many of the factors which prevent the lymphatic system from doing its job effectively fall within parental control.

In order to participate fully in a regime of recovery, it is necessary to understand the source of the problem. I have set out here to describe briefly and simply the functions and malfunctions of the lymph system, and to explain – in terms of this system – the difference between health and sickness. In so doing, it is my hope that this book will shed light on a little known but vital aspect of our bodies and health.

GETTING WELL, STAYING WELL

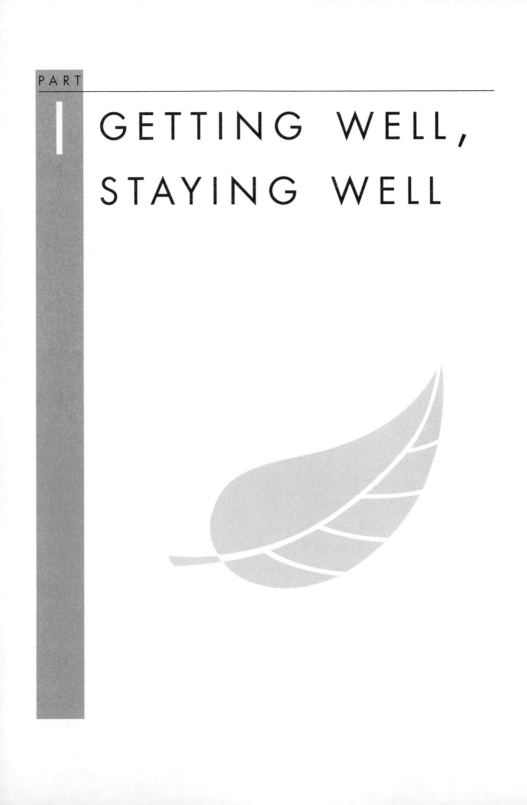

1 YOUR BODY'S FIRST LINE OF DEFENCE

What do all these people have in common?

> My daughter, Hannah, developed a small patch of eczema on the back of her knees when she was about six months old, but it was only really noticeable when she had a cold. After I stopped breastfeeding her at around nine months, it got much worse and I wondered whether the cow's milk might have something to do with it. By the time she was two, it was on her elbows, her thighs, her tummy and behind her ears. It looked very red and raw, especially behind her knees.
>
> The nights were the worst. It itched like mad and I just could not stop her from scratching, which made it bleed. She used to wake exhausted in the mornings and find it a real struggle to get through the day. People started to stare at her, too, and keep their distance as though she had some contagious disease, which really upset me and made her very self-conscious.

Jane, 34

> I used to suffer from the most terrible cystitis. It ruled my life. Apart from the excruciating pain of passing urine, when it was bad I just did not want to leave the house. If I did go out, I had to know that I was never more than a few minutes away from a lavatory. Long journeys were completely out of the question, and even going to a film became an ordeal. When I needed to go, I just couldn't hold on and the urge could return within minutes. It made me feel very low. My doctor had given me antibiotics on several occasions to get rid of the infection, but the cystitis always returned.

Catherine, 37

We got so used to our son, Nicholas, being slightly under the weather as a small child that we accepted it as normal. He was a very snuffly baby and picked up virtually every cold that was going. Then, around the age of seven, he started getting these really bad sore throats and high temperatures. He was always prescribed antibiotics by our doctor, which seemed to make him better, but within a couple of months he would go down with another sore throat and he was finding it harder and harder to shake them off. He was a real handful at home and his teachers were starting to complain about his behaviour at school as well. For some reason he seemed to find it really difficult to concentrate. The awful thing was, we just felt as though he was going downhill and had no idea what to do about it.

Joelle, 33

When I started out on my career as a professional singer I used to lose my voice so often that I did not dare to put myself up for solo roles. I would breathe a sigh of relief if my voice held out for auditions and was happy to settle for a place in the chorus, because I told myself that, if my voice did go, I could always get by mouthing the words.

Michael, 35

For as long as I can remember I seem to have had a permanent cold or a blocked nose, so that for a long time I had to breathe through my mouth and I snored so loudly at night that it used to wake my sister, who shared my room. When I was 10 my parents took me to see a specialist who said that my adenoids were causing the problem, and so I had them removed. The only difference after the operation was that I could breathe through my nose for the first time, but I still get sore throats all the time and seem to feel tired for no reason. I have also been doing really badly at school.

Emily, 17

All of these people are suffering from complaints arising from a breakdown in their lymphatic system – the body's Number 1 disease-fighting mechanism.

THE KEY TO GOOD HEALTH

The lymphatic network has two main functions: it acts as our body's combined sewage and drainage system and, at the same time, as its front line of defence. In other words, it works round the clock, vacuuming up debris and foreign bodies, removing excess fluids, fighting infection and repairing damage in every nook and cranny of the body.

Alongside the system of arteries, veins and capillaries which transports blood from our heart to our cells and back again, there is a separate – but connected – network of lymphatic channels. Unlike the arteries and veins, though, the lymphatic ducts open directly into the tissue spaces in between the cells. In the event of an infection, this allows them to carry away excess tissue fluids as well as minute foreign bodies such as bacteria.

Lymph is the name given to the fluid that passes along the lymphatic vessels towards the nearest group of lymph nodes, so that any dead cells, foreign or toxic substances can be filtered out and destroyed by the white blood cells before the fluid is returned to the veins.

Each set of lymph nodes is responsible for draining a particular area of the body, and are strategically placed around the body to act as centres for the production of antibodies against invading bacteria or viruses carried to them from the tissue spaces. The lymph nodes are helped by a small number of critical lymphatic structures – the tonsils, the adenoids, the appendix and the spleen. The first three form the body's first line of defence against infection by manufacturing antibodies in their own 'test tubes', capable of giving specific advanced protection against a range of 'bugs' that may invade in the future. The spleen is a huge lymph node and has a huge reserve of white cells to combat any infection.

Most people are barely aware of the existence of the lymphatic system within their own body, but it is a vital mechanism, and when it goes wrong it causes many health problems within the body.

Distressing conditions such as asthma, eczema, sinus trouble and cystitis are all caused by breakdowns in the smooth running of the lymphatic system. So too are many other debilitating ailments including bronchitis, laryngitis, arthritis, ear and eye problems. In other words, trouble within the lymphatic system can trigger a whole range of apparently unrelated complaints. Equally, as soon as the mechanism is restored to full working order, the symptoms can often be greatly or completely relieved.

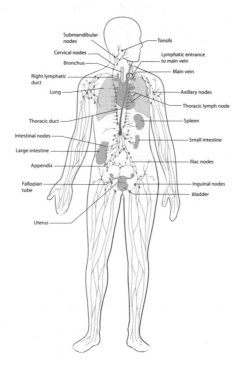

▲ THE LYMPHATIC SYSTEM

Under every big city lies a network of ducts, pipes and tunnels – unseen and largely unappreciated – which is vital to the health and survival of the city. While these networks are often triumphs of engineering, they are clumsy and primitive compared to the body's own, quite remarkable system of waste disposal – the lymphatic system.

The lymphatic system consists of tubes, filters, detoxicating units and chemical warfare plants of breathtaking complexity and efficiency.

Like any sophisticated mechanism, the lymphatic system needs careful maintenance if it is to maintain health and heal disease. Sadly, however, it is rarely given the attention it deserves and is all too often overlooked and abused. Because of its unobtrusive role, it is seldom considered as a possible cause when illness strikes the body.

OBSTACLES TO GOOD HEALTH

Under ideal conditions, the lymphatic system is an extremely efficient mechanism for dealing with infection rapidly, completely and often permanently. However, 'advances' in our way of life since primitive times, such as wearing clothes, using central heating and processing our food, have had the effect of weakening our lymphatic system. Huge population numbers also mean that we are regularly exposed to a greater number of high-grade infections than our systems were originally designed to cope with. Under these conditions, when greater demands are being placed on it, the efficient working of the lymphatic system can easily be undermined.

When the lymph nodes become overloaded with infection and debris, they begin to silt up. This slows down the passage of lymph through the nodes and causes back-pressure of fluid in the lymphatic vessels. The results are:

- reduced ability to resist and overcome infection
- an accumulation of fluid, causing swollen membranes which in the case of ducts obstruct the passages they line (e.g. from the sinuses and the middle ear)
- asthma

Some symptoms of an overburdened lymphatic system, such as constant infections, sore throats and bronchial troubles, may be obvious, but others are not usually associated with illness. A bad-tempered, inattentive and rude child, for example, may be punished for disruptive behaviour when what he really needs is treatment to his defective lymph nodes.

Early Warning System

Problems with the lymphatic system usually start at a very young age, although in some cases the main symptoms do not show up until much later in life. Some diseases, such as asthma, are considered hereditary and parents all too often resign themselves to the fact that their child will suffer – but this need not be so. Certainly, a child may have a tendency to the disease, but that can almost always be overcome by taking preventative action early in life and, where appropriate, carrying out simple massage techniques to maintain effective lymphatic drainage in the affected areas.

LYMPHATIC DRAINAGE TREATMENT

There is little place in my approach for the drugs which are commonly used by doctors to treat the ailments caused by lymphatic breakdown. The mainstay of my treatment involves 'physical' medicine – massage, ultrasonic waves and electrical muscle stimulation – to break up the debris and improve the flow of fluid through the lymph nodes, much as you would use a rubber plunger to clear tea-leaves that have blocked the wastepipe that drains your sink. Once the congestion in the nodes has been relieved and the drainage from the tissues improved, infections can be dealt with properly by the lymphatic system. As a result, the patient not only feels better, but is less likely to succumb to the next 'bug' that comes around.

In situations where home-based measures are not sufficient to treat the problem, it will be necessary to seek professional help. **The equipment and knowledge required to carry out the treatment that I recommend should be available from any reputable physiotherapist.**

The Treatment section of this book provides all the necessary guidelines for a professional therapist to follow. However, it is important to realize that there can come a time when the system breaks down irretrievably, at which point lymphatic drainage treatment, in any form, is not enough. This applies particularly to the tonsils and appendix, which can be destroyed by the bacteria they are trying to eliminate and become health hazards in themselves.

2 A GUIDE TO THE LYMPHATIC SYSTEM

HOW IT ALL BEGAN

We can trace the origins of the lymphatic system back millions of years, to when life started as primitive cells in the sea. These cells were totally dependent on their environment – extracting oxygen and food from the sea water and excreting their waste products into it. At a later stage of evolution, organisms probably developed a system of tubes which could take sea water into the more distant layers of cells and carry away waste products. This bypassed the need for each cell to have direct access to the sea, enabling organisms to be much larger.

Eventually, a 'closed' system of pipes developed, containing fluid which could take oxygen and food to every cell at any distance from the surface. Although an improvement in design terms, it still had a fault: if the protective surface of the organism was ruptured and invaders were able to get in, then the circulation would allow these predators unlimited access, thereby placing the organism under threat.

A new design was needed. This took the shape of the more sophisticated closed circulatory system that we have in our bodies today, which protects our network of arteries and veins from contamination by debris, foreign bodies and invading organisms. On the relatively rare occasions when bacteria or viruses do make their way into our tissue spaces, the means provided for their safe removal and eventual disposal is the lymphatic system.

CIRCULATION

Blood is pumped away by the heart, through the arteries and capillaries, to the tissues. At this point the clear fluid part of the blood – known as tissue fluid – diffuses from the capillaries into the tissue spaces, taking with it essential supplies of food, building materials and oxygen to nourish the surrounding tissues. It then diffuses back into the bloodstream through the walls at the other end of the capillaries, carrying with it carbon dioxide and waste products. The blood transporting these by-products then starts its return journey to the heart by means of the muscle pump. Every time a muscle contracts, it squeezes tissue fluid out of the muscle and nearby tissues, into the veins and fluid in the veins, back to the heart. Non-return valves ensure the flow is to the heart only. Nearby tissues also depend on adjacent muscles for their proper circulation.

The muscle contractions also have the same effect in promoting the lymphatic drainage.

BODY FLUIDS EXPLAINED

Blood is a complex fluid containing both red and white cells, as well as other substances such as salts and antibodies.

The red cells exchange oxygen from the lungs with carbon dioxide from the tissues.

The white cells, which include lymphocytes, are the scavengers and soldiers of the body whose job it is to protect the body against infection and fight infection when it occurs.

The white cells are carried by the blood to the site of any trouble, where they can engulf foreign bodies, bacteria or viruses.

Tissue fluid is basically blood without the red cells. When this fluid diffuses from the blood vessels into the tissue spaces, it carries with it white cells which may be needed to dispose of invaders.

UNDER ATTACK

Every minute of each day the tissue spaces are under siege from a variety of unwanted foreign bodies. These include:

- the remnants of dead, damaged or bruised cells
- particles which enter through damaged skin
- bacteria and viruses which we breathe in from the air or take in by mouth

The skin normally acts as an impenetrable barrier against invaders from outside. However, the smallest graze or cut can provide an opening for bacteria to enter. The skin can also be penetrated by injections of poisonous substances from the stings and bites of insects, parasites, snakes and other creatures – or from fungi which grow on the skin, such as athlete's foot.

Often, disease-causing bacteria and viruses are found in minute droplets of mucus coughed or sneezed into the air by other creatures. Undesirable bacteria and viruses may also find their way into the body through contaminated food and drink. These invading organisms then multiply rapidly to spread disease. Those injected by other organisms such as mosquitoes, however, are often less easily overcome and eliminated.

THE LYMPHATIC SYSTEM FIGHTS BACK

Our body's most powerful tool for dealing with the threat posed by insidious invaders is, without question, the lymphatic system. Like an efficient police force, the lymphatic system corners and captures any invaders, or removes them to a place where they can be sorted out quickly, effectively and permanently.

If the skin is penetrated and a tissue space invaded, nature has several defence mechanisms to call upon:

- an increase in the blood supply to the affected area in order to provide more nourishment, antibodies and more fighting white cells

- the secretion of large amounts of mucus by the mucous glands, found in the throat, nose, sinuses, ears and appendix (which normally keep the delicate membranes healthily moist), designed to wash away the offending infection or irritant and to act as a mild antiseptic

- pre-formed antibodies in the tissue fluid, which work on the invaders in order to stem the invasion until more powerful reinforcements from the immune system can be manufactured and brought into play

- in some areas, if the infection is not dealt with quickly the body tries to wall it off with fibrous tissue, creating a pocket of infection, such as a boil. In other areas, like the abdominal or lung cavity, the membrane lining becomes sticky and may attach itself to nearby surfaces to contain the infection.

THE LYMPH NODES

There are eight main groups of lymph nodes, each responsible for draining its own particular area of the body (see diagram).

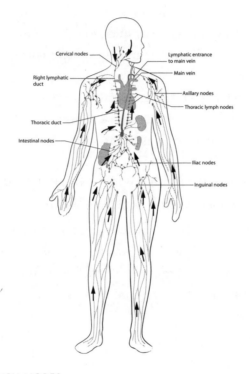

Cervical nodes

Lymphatic entrance to main vein

Main vein

Right lymphatic duct

Axillary nodes

Thoracic lymph nodes

Thoracic duct

Intestinal nodes

Iliac nodes

Inguinal nodes

▲ THE LYMPH NODES

The body has been designed so that it contains a great deal of equipment in a very small space. As part of this space-saving design, the lymph nodes have been given the job of draining a number of otherwise unconnected parts of the body.

Lymph nodes act as:

- filters
- waste disposal units like those found in sinks
- detoxicating units
- factories producing powerful chemicals.

In their role as waste disposal units, the lymph nodes filter out any impurities in the lymph and then reduce everything to a soluble form, so it can be safely returned to the bloodstream to be transported for excretion or disposal by the liver, kidneys or bowel.

The process is rather like the sewage system for a group of houses in a village. Each house has its own sewage pipe which leads into one big pipe at the end of the village and, eventually, flows into the river. The sewage goes through a series of detoxicating and liquidizing stations, so that, by the time it reaches the river – the equivalent of returning to the bloodstream – everything that was harmful has been made safe and there are no solids left.

Each lymph node is also a factory unit composed of a vast network of cells capable of producing a type of white blood cell called a *lymphocyte*. These lymphocytes have the job of sizing up each invader (called an antigen), and then manufacturing a chemical (called an antibody) which is designed to wipe out that particular enemy. The antibodies pass from the lymph to the bloodstream, and so to the invaded tissue spaces, where they coagulate (engulf) the enemy. As soon as enough antibodies are formed, they set about disposing of all the foreign organisms. This is the most decisive way of overcoming infection.

ANTIBODIES

Antibodies are formed only against **unwanted** organisms that invade the tissues and end up in the lymph system. We have a large variety of harmless and even useful bacteria which live on our skin, in our mouths, down our breathing tubes and, most important of all, in our intestines. These bacteria carry out many essential processes that the body cannot perform for itself, and also manufacture some vital substances. We rely on these bacteria for good health, so it is essential that the body can distinguish between 'good' and 'bad' bacteria.

Fluid that contains a motley collection of bacteria or viruses, white cells (which may have engulfed invaders), other debris and any undesirable chemicals present in the tissue spaces is washed down special tubes or ducts, known as lymph vessels or lymphatics. It moves through the lymph ducts to the nearest cluster of lymph nodes or glands. So lymph is actually tissue fluid when it gets into the lymphatic vessels.

LYMPHATIC OVERLOAD

Healthy lymph nodes (commonly referred to as 'glands') are soft and not easily felt. However, if the area they are responsible for draining has been taken over by an infection, then the additional fluid and debris will cause them to swell and become more prominent. The nodes increase in size as the fluid drains through, leaving behind solid particles. If the problem persists, they enlarge still further to cope with the extra workload, in the same way that a manufacturer might expand the size of his factory to meet increased orders.

Chronically congested lymph nodes will usually feel hard to the touch as well.

It is easy to see why swollen lymph nodes are such a useful diagnostic tool for a doctor trying to ascertain whether a patient, particularly a child, has an infection. An ear infection, for example, will cause the lymph nodes in the neck – which drain the ear – to expand, while infections in the foot or leg will give rise to swellings in the groin, and an infected finger may result in tender lumps under the arm.

Harry, aged nine, pricked his finger with a rose thorn when he was helping his mother in the rose garden. The thorn broke off and became lodged in his finger, but he did not want to tell his mother because he was afraid she might be cross, so he left it there overnight. The next morning it was so painful that he owned up and his mother put antiseptic on his finger. Despite this, it became steadily worse. The area around the thorn was very red and angry and there were red streaks going up his arm.

His mother, now quite worried, took Harry to the doctor. The doctor examined his finger and felt under his armpit, where she found some enlarged and tender lymph nodes. The infection had reached quite a serious point, in the sense that the bacteria had not only made a successful invasion where the thorn had ruptured the skin, but had also travelled up the lymph ducts, inflaming them – hence the red streaks – and the lymph nodes as well.

The doctor removed the thorn and some pus, and put Harry onto antibiotics to eliminate the infection before it made its way into the bloodstream, where it might have caused septicaemia. Fortunately, it all cleared up fairly quickly and, as soon as Harry's finger was better, the swelling in the lymph nodes subsided.

OPERATION LYMPH

The lymphatic system is like a strategically placed army with numerous garrisons all over the body. In the areas most likely to be invaded there are many patches of lymph tissue. This is why the thin membranes needed to line the nose, mouth, intestine and breathing apparatus are especially well protected, rather like a series of forts on a frontier.

If the invading organism should penetrate the outermost defences, it will soon come up against more powerful strongholds – the lymph nodes. And, in the forefront, ready to provide ultimate back-up to a beleaguered army, there are a few large and strategically located 'castles': the tonsils, adenoids, appendix, Peyer's patches throughout the bowel and, the giant of them all, the spleen.

These scattered clusters of lymph tissue form a network around the body. If one mode stops working properly then another will cover. If that fails, another will take over, and so on.

DEFENCE WEAPONS

The tonsils, adenoids and appendix are all vital lymph complexes which are activated to repel organisms entering the body through the mouth or nose, and in the food or drink that we consume. They also act as an advance defence mechanism against these everyday bacteria.

The lymph system is not equally divided on either side of the body. It has a very small catchment area on the top right side of the body, and a huge network that drains everywhere else. This may explain why many lymphatic complaints are left-sided and why blockages are more likely to occur on that side of the body. In the lower three-quarters of the body, the lymph ducts that drain the legs, abdomen and chest all run together to form a large vessel called the thoracic duct. Both sides of the system ultimately feed into big veins located just below the collarbone which carry blood back to the heart.

TONSILS AND ADENOIDS

We are born with six tonsils: two at the root of our tongue, two at the side of our throat and two nasal tonsils, called the adenoids, in the back of our nose where the nasal opening joins the throat.

Each tonsil measures about two centimetres square and is enclosed in a close-fitting bag, rather like a precious stone in its setting (see diagram, page 63).

Tonsils are in fact large collections of lymph tissue and carry out the same functions as other lymph nodes in the body. In primitive times, when we scavenged for our food and would often have had to content ourselves with the putrid leftovers of other hunters, the tonsils had to deal with a continuous stream of different kinds of bacteria. For this reason, we have a particularly generous blood supply to our throat and there is a great deal of lymphoid tissue in the surrounding membranes, providing healthy tonsils with an amazing capacity to cope with a barrage of organisms.

Tonsils have little recesses on their surface, where bacteria enter and are cultured by the tonsil. The tonsil then manufactures antibodies against those particular organisms to enable it to provide a high level of immunity as fast as possible in the event of an attack. Even if they are not immediately required, the antibodies remain in the blood and diffuse into the tissue fluids so they can spring into action should that particular organism invade again at some later stage.

Some families of invading organisms share antibodies, which means that any member of that family can be partly immobilized by the antibodies generated against the original invader. Babies are born with their mother's antibodies in their circulation. Colostrum, which breastfed babies receive during their first 48 hours, is a further invaluable source of antibodies which provides them with vital protection during their early months.

A child is likely to come into contact with – and so form antibodies against – virtually all the common bacteria that he or she is ever likely to meet by the age of six or seven. It is during this phase of life that the tonsils and appendix serve their most useful purpose.

Tonsils have to work incredibly hard – whether they are dealing with a series of minor infections or repelling one acute attack. In the process they will, like all lymph nodes, increase in size in order to manufacture more antibodies and deal more effectively with the infection. A child who has suffered recurrent throat infections will probably have very enlarged tonsils. This is not a reason in itself to have them removed, as it usually means they are doing their job. If, however, there are signs that enlarged tonsils are infected (see page 69 for guidelines), then they should definitely be removed.

Nature has provided us with such a good back-up defence system that if the tonsils are removed at an age when the body still requires a lot of immunity, one of the other groups of lymph nodes in that area will immediately step in and take over. You may be surprised to learn that you have many clusters of lymph tissue all over your tongue and at the back of your throat which are capable of growing to replace a missing but necessary tonsil.

Julie was 19 and not at all well when I first saw her. Apparently she had begun suffering from intermittent infections even at the tender age of nine months; by the time she was three, she was constantly troubled by sore throats and ear trouble. When she was six she had her tonsils removed and, although this was followed by an initial improvement, within a few years her throat trouble had returned and continued ever since. She felt tired and generally unwell.

On examination I saw that there were two reasonably sized tonsils present in her throat. The membranes lining the throat contain a great deal of lymph tissue; parts of this had obviously regrown to form new tonsils to replace the damaged ones that had been removed at a time when they were still needed. However, these too had become infected, probably because the lymph nodes draining them had become partly blocked as a result of the infection in the first tonsils. Once the second set of tonsils were removed, Julie's health improved dramatically.

THE APPENDIX

The appendix is a small tube situated at the end of a short sac called the caecum, which is connected to the large bowel. The caecum carries a store of bacteria which are useful in breaking down some parts of vegetables, most notably the tough cellulose, which the ordinary digestive system cannot dissolve. As humans are really designed to eat meat, the caecum is very rudimentary compared to the mechanism you would find in a plant-eating animal such as a cow.

The whole of the outer surface of the bowel and the inner surface of the abdominal cavity is lined by a protective membrane called the peritoneum, which houses many of the blood vessels, lymphatic vessels and lymph nodes serving the bowel.

The appendix is the largest of a huge number of patches of lymph tissue in the bowel, and acts with them as the first line of defence against infections occurring in that area.

In much the same way that the tonsils deal with infections of the mouth and nose, the appendix takes in the bacteria that live in the bowel and cultures them to form antibodies against them. This ensures that you always have in your blood a high concentration of antibodies against most bacteria that are likely to affect or infect you. This gives the body a head start in any severe infection.

As with the tonsils, by the time you are around seven years old, the appendix will have formed some protection against most of the bacteria which are likely to invade your bowel. After the age of 10 it has little real value, and by the age of around 14 it usually becomes largely inactive.

THE SPLEEN

The spleen is a large spongy organ located in the upper left side of the abdomen near the stomach, which has much in common with the lymph nodes. It is packed with lymphocytes and is the body's greatest producer of antibodies. This means that, if the spleen ever has to be removed for any reason, resistance to infection becomes dangerously reduced.

3 BREAKDOWN AND REPAIR

We have seen the critical part that the lymphatic system plays in the body's defence mechanism and immune system as a whole, and how it can help us to resist and overcome infection. No less important is its caretaking role, which involves maintaining healthy conditions in the tissues of the body – ensuring that they are properly drained and free of any unnecessary debris, so that illness is less likely to occur.

A useful analogy is to compare the process of lymphatic drainage with the sewage pipes for a row of houses, the toilets in each house representing the various tissues drained by a lymph node, and the lymph node akin to an inspection manhole where blockages might occur.

In normal circumstances, this system would act efficiently and be able to cope with fairly heavy demands. Under certain conditions, however, the drainage process might slow down or grind to a complete halt, possibly due to damage in the soil pipe itself. A more common occurrence is for the system to be affected either by a constant influx of debris from the toilets which slowly and by degrees starts to block the inspection pit, or by a sudden barrage of items from one toilet that obstructs it more or less instantly.

In the case of the lymphatic system, partial blockage of the nodes is usually brought about by a series of low-grade infections, such as occur in the bladder or the throat, by one continuous very low-grade infection like athlete's foot, or else by a very intense infection, say in the throat or lung.

It is important to understand that the lymph nodes do not become obstructed on their own. Blockage is always caused by the debris arising from infections brought into them by the lymph. A series of minor sore throats or one particularly virulent throat infection, for example, may overload the lymph nodes in the neck which drain the throat. In their capacity as filters, these nodes then become partially blocked.

Just as a blocked drain will cause the offending toilet to overflow as well as some or all the other ones in the street connected to the same system, so a congested lymph node will prevent the tissue fluid from draining, causing the tissues to swell and upsetting tissue circulation in the catchment area. Operations or injuries, particularly in the neck area, may involve damage to lymph ducts, which can upset the proper drainage through these channels. Although the body may grow new lymph vessels, the effects of the initial blockage need to be addressed to avoid longer-term problems.

SWOLLEN MEMBRANES – EASY ACCESS

Healthy membranes are unimaginably thin, being only one square flat cell thick. These are 'pavement cells', so called because they resemble the stone slabs of a pavement. In adverse circumstances, however, these cells multiply on top of each other, thickening the membranes to (relatively speaking) massive proportions.

Sluggish tissue circulation does not provide cells with enough nourishment. In their weakened state, the cells multiply to form a thick wall between the bacteria invading from the outside and the tissues. A good example of this is the area at the back of the throat. As the membranes swell, the soft palate becomes soggy and thickens up – instead of being taut and lying flat – and we find ourselves with a snoring problem.

This enlarged wall is intended to provide increased protection, but has the opposite effect because the outside layer of the membrane is further removed from the protection of defenders and nutrients in the tissue circulation. As the army of white cells is prevented from reaching the bacteria, it is unable to do its work to immobilize them so they can be carried away in the lymph vessels. Instead, the bacteria take refuge in the outer part of the thick wall, and start to multiply.

The increased distance between the tissue fluid and the invading bacteria also means that the antibody response is not activated and, with such short supplies of weapons (i.e. white cells), the membrane is even less able to cope with the infection and throw it off. If a castle were under prolonged attack, the defenders could build an ever-thicker wall to improve security. It could become half a mile thick. This would be very counterproductive, however, as the enemy could climb it unseen and regroup on top of the wall, ready for a major assault.

The situation is compounded as attacks by bacteria or viruses become more frequent, which, in turn speeds up the blockage of the lymph nodes, weakening still further the antibody response.

We have already seen how several seemingly unconnected areas can be drained by the same lymph nodes, and that the back-pressure of fluid caused by a partial blockage can spread up the tubes leading to other parts of the body, to affect the drainage from other membranes. An irritation in the throat could, for example, affect the drainage from the sinuses or middle ear. In such a situation, these membranes would also thicken, making them vulnerable to attack by any bacteria or viruses that settle in that area. The congestion will also bring with it a range of other specific problems such as the allergic response that triggers an attack of hay fever.

The general consequences of lymphatic breakdown for our health include:

- a reduced antibody response and reduced ability to resist and recover from infection
- a weakened repair mechanism so that any operations, cuts or wounds will take longer to heal
- an accumulation of excess fluid causing swelling, particularly in the face, ankles and hands
- the thickening of the lining of drains causing obstruction from such obstructions as the middle ear or sinuses.

The conventional way to treat an infection is to bring in extra weapons from outside, such as antibiotics, to help the failing army win the battle. The disadvantage of this method is that it encourages the army to become sloppy about maintaining its equipment, and complacent in the event of any future crisis. It may also make less powerful enemies more likely to attack as they see the rundown state of the defences.

HELPING THE BODY TO HEAL ITSELF

My approach is to enable the body to look after its own defence unaided, by rectifying internal problems so that it is not only able to cope with a particular emergency, but will be much more effective in a future crisis. Moreover, its very strength will act as a major deterrent to aggressors.

The treatment I recommend aims to improve the drainage of the tissue fluid through the lymph sewers, thereby reducing the overflow or 'traffic jam' in the tissue spaces. This promotes healthy tissue circulation and alleviates swollen membranes, with immediate benefits for the existing complaint and better prospects for the future health of the individual.

Once the lymph nodes are operating effectively:

- the health of the tissues themselves improves
- dead cells, bacteria and debris can be cleared and disposed of
- the supply of white cells and antibodies to the area returns to normal
- drainage tubes are cleared.

TREATMENT

The treatment required to restore lymphatic circulation and drainage involves several forms of 'physical' medicine determined by the particular complaint and the accessibility of the area concerned. In most cases, the affected part of the body can be treated, as well as the remote part of the associated drainage system. However, in certain instances, such as problems affecting the remote middle and inner ear, only the drainage system can be accessed.

The treatment uses a modified version of conventional physiotherapy techniques and should therefore be available from any qualified physiotherapist.

It can involve any or all of the following (see Treatment section beginning on page 50 for full details):

- Massage to decongest and improve the function of the lymph nodes. The massage need last only a few minutes and is a straightforward process that can easily be carried out at home – on yourself, on your child or on another adult – with huge benefits.
- Ultrasound to disperse blockages and encourage the healing of damaged tissues.
- Electrical muscle stimulation – to assist lymphatic flow and drainage by making the muscles in the affected area contract and relax rhythmically as a whole group.

> Simple massage techniques are extremely effective and can achieve the same end result in the majority of cases as mechanical techniques – without the need for professional help – over a slightly longer time span.

People vary enormously in the number of treatments they require. This depends not only on the severity of the problem and the physical make-up of the patient, but also on the skill of the therapist. There is usually a significant improvement early on in the treatment, but patients may need anything between 5 and 20 sessions to reduce the clinical signs to an acceptable level. After this, symptoms may still take several months to resolve fully. This applies especially to swollen membranes, which may have become many thousands of times their normal thickness.

Drugs can be a useful back-up to this physical medicine. In painful conditions produced by an inflammatory process, anti-inflammatory drugs help by significantly reducing the level of prostaglandin, a substance secreted locally in the tissues which is designed to bolster the tissues' ability to cope with any emergency, but which can in itself prove harmful if produced, as it so often is, excessively.

4 HELPING YOUR BODY TO HELP ITSELF

Exercise, Fresh Air and A Healthy Diet

It took a million years for human beings to evolve and exist in the conditions of primitive society. Civilization has turned almost every facet of this existence upside down, so any assistance we can provide to help our bodies to cope with the very artificial circumstances of our present lifestyle must be worthwhile.

THE DOUBLE-SIDED COIN

We so take for granted modern civilization, with our houses and clothes to protect us from the elements and the food industry to provide us with safe things to eat and drink, that it may come as quite a shock to many people to find that these 'advances' are actually the cause of many of our most common and persistent health problems.

From the first months of life, huge demands are placed on a baby's lymphatic system, which must work hard to fight every germ that comes its way and produce antibodies for future protection. A small baby has a huge lymphatic system in relation to its tiny body, but the lymph nodes are still very small compared to those of an adult, whereas the bacteria, viruses and dead cells are all full-sized. For this reason it is considerably easier for the lymph nodes of the very young to become congested.

A BARRAGE OF INFECTION

From a very early age we are subjected to a greater degree of airborne infection than nature intended. In primitive days, people wandered about in small groups. As with other natural herds or packs, there was probably no interaction between these groupings. There would have been few young children in each group, and so a minimum of contact with new infection.

Nowadays, babies go about in prams and are admired by an endless stream of people. Then there are shops, supermarkets, playgroups, parties, bus rides and holidays – all potentially bringing babies into contact with a huge diversity of infection. Hardly a day passes when a child does not come into close proximity with another child or strange adult who might pass on a germ through a touch, a cough or a sneeze.

There is every reason to believe that we can maintain our health despite the impact of our civilized lifestyle, provided we use our bodies to the full and keep them in optimum condition by keeping **as near as possible to the conditions for which our bodies were designed**.

KEEP ON MOVING

With the exception of professional sportspeople, our present lifestyle is extremely sedentary compared to primitive days, when we would have been continually on the move. This has serious implications for our health, since the lymphatic system, which has no central pump like the heart to power it, relies almost exclusively on the regular milking action of the muscles to drive fluid out of the tissue spaces and through the network of lymphatic vessels back to the heart.

If you spend the majority of your time sitting or standing and rarely break out of a walk, then your muscle pump will be insufficiently activated to maintain your lymphatic circulation at a level which promotes good health. As the mechanism is used less frequently, the drainage becomes less effective and excess fluid and waste products start to accumulate in the tissue spaces, creating the ideal conditions for disease to develop – and thus the potential for blockages in the lymph nodes. It is therefore vitally important that you take time each day to get all your muscles moving in order to keep your tissues healthy.

Everyone who does regular exercise acknowledges that they feel a lot better for it. Once you are aware of the benefits – which are impossible to overstate – it is a question of regarding exercise as a habit that you need to develop. In terms of lymphatic drainage, gentle rhythmical forms of exercise such as swimming, aqua-aerobics and Pilates are particularly effective. Rebounding on a mini-trampoline can give a massive boost to lymphatic circulation because of the constant shifts in internal pressure created as your body is suspended weightless in mid-air and then makes contact with the springy mat of the trampoline.

Good breathing habits and full use of your lung capacity will also help to maintain a healthy flow of lymphatic fluid (see page 114 ['Asthma' section] for breathing exercises). This is because the pumping of air in and out of the lungs also changes the pressures inside the chest and this 'pulls' fluid (blood and lymph) in vessels into the chest and then pushes it into the heart.

It is important to remember that the moment you have anything wrong with your body, fluid will automatically collect in that part. You are undermining your ability to cope with more chronic illness if you allow yourself to become too sedentary. Many people who come to me with back pain say that they were once very active but their circumstances have changed and they no longer have time for exercise. After six months of this new way of life, they suddenly suffer a lot of back pain. This is frequently due to sluggish tissue circulation causing a gradual build-up of waste products in the tissue spaces of the back.

Exercise produces a large quantity of heat, so it is the healthiest way to keep warm without resorting to extra layers of clothing or relying heavily on external forms of heating. Active children, who always prefer to be lightly dressed, should be our role models in this respect. Needless to say, if you sit still for long periods of time you will feel the cold much more than someone who is permanently on the move.

In children, it is the lymphatic system of the throat and lungs that causes problems. The rest of the system is rarely challenged until later in life. To explain why children are so vulnerable to constant colds and throat infections – and to enable parents and teachers to play an active part in children's healthcare – we need to look at the way the body reacts to changes in its environment, especially temperature.

A BREATH OF FRESH AIR

All engines – the human body included – require an effective cooling mechanism to enable them to dispose of the waste heat that they generate. Many animals have solved the problem of dissipating the considerable heat produced by muscular activity by panting air. They have a very large blood supply to the nose and throat, so the action of panting has the effect of cooling down the blood – and therefore the body as a whole. Elephants have large ears to act as radiators, but this is inadequate in the heat of the day, when they roll in water or mud, coating their skin to cool down.

When humans developed muscles that could continue working for long periods, the amount of heat generated was greatly in excess of the cooling ability of the throat mechanism. So we shed our fur to make available the huge area of the skin for cooling to replace the throat.

This cooling effect was increased still further by the evaporation of fluid through sweating. This means that humans, by varying the supply of blood and sweat to the skin, are able to maintain a constant body temperature over a wide variation in both external heat and muscular effort.

If this mechanism were allowed to develop fully of its own accord, then no clothes would be needed to maintain normal body temperature under practically all conditions. There is the true story of a Sherpa who, dressed in only his loincloth on an expedition well above the snow line in the Himalayas, was offered a suit of clothing on the grounds that he must be feeling the cold. He refused it, saying that his whole body, like our face, was never covered and did not feel the cold.

OVERHEATING OR OVERCLOTHING?

While newborns are unable to control their body temperature, clearly older babies require help only with extremes of temperature, otherwise the human race could not have survived. Because of their vulnerability, infants are provided with a thick layer of fat to insulate them from loss of heat, including around the hands and feet. As they become mobile and start to run around, generating more internal warmth, they lose this fat.

As soon as we start putting 'fur' back on our children, with layers of clothing, fleece-lined body suits and piles of warm blankets, their bodies are no longer able to cool down in the way that nature intended, and such children are likely to become overheated. In reaction, the body – the heat-diffusing mechanism of the skin having failed – makes a desperate attempt to go back to the throat, the old system of cooling down.

In nature, when a new set-up replaces an older or less efficient one, the original one is often retained, but may be converted to a different use. If the new system is demolished or impaired, then nature tries to re-instate the old one to do the job. Unfortunately, however, this system may not be able to revert to its original function.

So, the overclothed child – no longer able to cool himself adequately through the skin – falls back on a version of the primitive panting mechanism to control his body temperature. The body greatly increases the blood supply to the throat and tongue. However, without the capacity to exhale a large quantity of air (if we did, we would blow out too much carbon dioxide and upset our blood chemistry), the excessive fluid in the throat which comes with the increased circulation does not evaporate, which affects the child's health in the following ways:

- congestion in the membranes of the nose and throat
- reduced resistance and reduced ability to fight infection
- overloaded lymph nodes

It is always with the best intentions that parents overclothe their children, but in the interests of your child's health it is important to suppress your natural instinct to be overprotective. Children actually hate being too warm. There are so many occasions when I see children yelling as another blanket is piled on the pram, and then kicking in a desperate attempt to remove it. And yet this battle continues, ostensibly in the child's interest.

People often tell me that their children cry at night and no reason can be found. I can assure you that it is usually because they are too hot. Such children are nearly always sweaty and trying to get rid of their bedclothes. The answer is simply to remove most of the covers. When clothing is kept to an absolute minimum, the child is happier and the crying stops.

George's parents phoned to ask if I would come to the house to see him. They said that he was only 18 months old and had such bad asthma that he was too ill to travel. George's asthma attacks were indeed very bad and, whenever they seemed life-threatening, his parents resorted to an oxygen cylinder. George had been in hospital twice already.

I shall never forget visiting George. When I arrived at the house I was shown to his room. Although it was late spring, I was hit by a wall of heat as I walked through the door. His mum took me over to the cot and there, on top of the cot, was a fur eiderdown. Below that was a quilt and then three blankets and a sheet. Beneath this was a bundle of clothing several layers thick, which, once removed, finally revealed little George. He was absolutely soaking with sweat and had a rash on his neck and bottom.

I could hear a 'rattle' in his chest and, on feeling the lymph nodes in his neck, noticed they were already enlarged. There was also a tight feel to the muscles of the back, opposite the root of the lung. I tactfully explained to his mother that man had shed his fur to try and enable us to lose heat. By 'putting the fur back' onto George, the membranes of his nose and throat had become so swollen that fluid was pouring from them down to his lungs.

I told her that, as so young a child was largely unable to cough the mucus up, the only way of preventing the fluid from entering the lungs was by the tubes closing down in a spasm, which is how an asthma attack starts. I suggested that if she slowly started to reduce the layers of clothing and the heat in his room, and let some fresh air in, she would be taking some vital steps towards her son's recovery.

She understood what I was telling her and, three weeks later, she rang to say that George was so much better she wondered if she still needed to bring him for treatment. Remembering the enlarged lymph nodes, I suggested that she did so that I could check that everything was all right. In the end George had three treatments on his lymph nodes, and remained fit from then on.

Mothers often ask for guidelines about ideal levels of clothing. It is a difficult question to answer as every child has differing requirements: a plumper child probably loses less heat, but then a thinner child is probably more active and so generates more.

Children are far more likely to be upset by being overclothed than by being too cold. Layers of light clothing are the most comfortable and versatile way of controlling body temperature. If they are cold, they will soon let you know. When out of doors, my guide is to try to let your child do without a vest or a coat, even in winter, but carry an extra layer with you, just in case. You may well be surprised at how little your child actually needs in the way of extra clothing when he or she is running around outside.

To test a small child's body temperature, place a finger down the back of his or her neck. If it is warm, then your child is fine. There is no point in feeling hands and feet, as nature does not waste energy in keeping hands and feet warm when so much energy is needed for growing, playing and learning. In the very young, nature conveniently puts a thick layer of fat on fingers and feet – making them appealingly chubby – to insulate the inner person from the outside cold. If your child has very warm hands or feet, this means that the heat has got through all the fat insulation to the outside. That child is probably grossly overheated.

Habit plays an important part in your body's reaction to temperature, so it is wise to start instilling good habits at a young age. Temperature is relative – if you always wear too many clothes then you get to the point where you feel cold if you take your coat off!

POSITIVE IONS AND POLLUTION

It is a stock joke among doctors that, when people come home from a really healthy skiing holiday in a mountainous area with clean air, snow and sunshine, where they are exposed to negative ions, they catch flu on the plane home or during the first few days back, when they re-enter an atmosphere filled with positive ions. This is actually directly related to the charge of the ions in the air.

The body does not react to negatively charged particles in the atmosphere, as found in mountainous regions, and so its defence mechanism is not challenged by them and more or less switches off. That explains why, on leaving a country with such 'clean' air, the body is not prepared to fight off a new infection, perhaps passed on by a cough or sneeze on the aeroplane.

The air is filled with positively and negatively charged electrical particles known as ions. Positive ions are produced by air conditioning, central heating, the air we breathe out, chemical fumes and machinery and any turbulence. Positive ions increase dramatically before storms and with certain winds – and they attract each other. When positive ions predominate, we feel tired and unwell. The most positively charged wind in the Gobi desert is known as 'Arreal' – the angel of death.

An excess of negative ions, on the other hand – found in fresh seaside or mountain air and after a storm – improves both our physical and mental well-being.

In any country where houses are heated and pollution is rife, the air we inhale tends to be charged with positive ions. The body reacts badly to positively charged particles. If you breathe them in, they pass through the walls of your lungs into your blood and affect the platelets, causing them to produce excess quantities of a substance called serotonin.

Although serotonin is an important 'chemical messenger' mainly within the brain, excessive levels outside this in the body have the effect of increasing any existing swelling or inflammation and will therefore intensify any congestion around the nose and throat area, particularly in young children, and so aggravate any infection. Too much serotonin can also make you more susceptible to other infections.

The direct effect of positive ionization on health is well illustrated by one of my patients, 58-year-old Gladys, who noticed that her catarrhal condition altered with the weather. When the air was charged with positive ions her condition became dramatically worse.

Gladys had been catarrhal as a child and caught a lot of colds. From around the age of 30 she was bothered by a blocked nose and heavy catarrh, which had gradually become worse. She had an operation to have her sinuses washed out and had felt a lot better for some time afterwards. However, before long she suffered several attacks of really bad infection which had required antibiotics. Even at her best, she was grappling with a continuous, low-grade catarrhal condition.

One of the things that bothered Gladys most was how dramatically her condition varied with the weather. On nice, dry, sunny days she was relatively fine. However, even before the clouds started rolling in her catarrhal state would begin to intensify. She could actually predict in advance when the weather was going to break – or when it was going to improve – by the state of her health.

She had also noticed how often, especially in summer and autumn, the weather preceding a full moon was good and she felt well. Just about the time of the full moon, however, the weather tended to turn suddenly and her condition would deteriorate. She also observed how much worse she felt during the build-up to a thunderstorm. But, as soon as the storm broke and there were a few flashes of lightning to negatively charge the particles in the air around her, her condition improved.

Stale air is charged with excessive positive ions which can greatly diminish the body's ability to cope with everyday bugs. As we breathe out, we increase the positive ions in the air, so it is important to replace stale with fresh air to restore the balance. If you live in a house where the windows and doors are kept firmly shut and no draughts are allowed in, then the atmosphere will be heavily charged with positive ions. We all need exposure to fresh air. This is especially true of children, who should be encouraged to play outside as much as possible.

Warmed air is often stale air. All forms of heating give out positive ions. With open fires these ions are pulled up the chimney so they do not affect the atmosphere. However, other heaters tend to have a detrimental effect on the air in the room, increasing with the degree of turbulence. A fan heater produces a large number of positive ions; most of us feel instinctively that it is an uncomfortable form of heating.

Even worse are the effects of air conditioning. Circulating fans cause turbulence and, as air passes down ducts, it becomes more positively charged. In modern buildings where space is at a premium, ducts tend to be smaller and the speed of passage through them therefore greater. This markedly increases the rate of positive ionization and is probably the main cause of 'sick building syndrome' prevalent in office blocks.

Artificial heating or air conditioning is not a good environment for anyone to live or work in, and is certainly not healthy for children. I firmly believe that it is unnecessary to have any form of heating in a bedroom, and have already explained how overheating during the night can interfere with efficient lymphatic function in the same way as overclothing can during the day.

A number of the substances involved in urban pollution are in themselves irritating, such as smoke, grit, dust, soot from engine exhausts (especially diesel), factory smoke and certain gases. The very presence of pollution also makes more particles to increase the level of positive ions, and aggravates any existing inflammation and congestion thus obstructing passages and increasing levels of secretion. The treatment described in this book can help to reduce the adverse effects of pollution by restoring normal function to the membranes.

> With normal ventilation, the air in a room may be changed up to six or so times an hour, which means that you would need a negative ionizer of substantial size in order to keep up with the continual re-introduction of any positive ions being manufactured.

USE IT OR LOSE IT!

All the equipment in our body is only as strong as the demands we place on it. We have already noted the fact that our bodies pack a great deal of machinery into a small space. In accordance with this space-saving principle, we maintain and develop only those systems that are actually in use: if you were to put your arm in a sling for long enough, your muscles would gradually degenerate and eventually it would become useless. You have to use everything in your body to keep it going. The lymphatic system is no exception.

There is no doubt that frequent attacks of infection are needed to maintain a vigorous defence mechanism. Children insulated from all infection tend to be the very ones that seem to 'go down with everything', as they have weak immune systems and do not respond so vigorously when an infection strikes. Clearly, there are certain infections which it is best to avoid or protect your child against – such as measles, mumps, German measles, polio and tuberculosis – but, as a general rule, it is unwise to keep your child away from run-of-the-mill infections.

As with any other mechanism in your body, the lymphatic system can only provide a sufficient level of immunity if it is constantly exercised and challenged to build up its strength and resilience. If it is under-used or over-protected – either by being shielded from contact with other people who may be carrying an infection or by excessive caution over food and domestic hygiene – it will become weak and ineffectual.

In the same way, it is important not to be over-cautious about the bacteria in the food and drink we consume. Our primitive ancestors were scavengers as well as hunters and would eat almost anything – germs and all. In order to cope with this stream of bacteria, we developed a very effective defence mechanism, part of which involves manufacturing many antibodies in advance.

Nowadays we seem keen to use every method at our disposal to limit the number of bacteria coming into contact with our systems.

For example, food is sterilized and kept in fridges, both in shops and in homes, sell-by dates are imposed, additives are put in to prevent bacteria and fungi from growing, food is deep-frozen, often after sterilization, and fruit, vegetables and meat are stored in shrink wrappings or protected at all costs from the flies and wasps that would have been all over them 50 years ago. In fact, almost every aspect of domestic life is being sterilized in an attempt to wipe out infection.

I view with horror the increasing range of products – washing up liquids, dishcloths, chopping boards, etc. – which are impregnated with anti-bacterial substances. The more we sterilize everything and try to eliminate bacteria from every morsel we eat, the more susceptible we become to milder and milder bacteria and viruses. These days, people are constantly going down with one 'bug' after another – in my youth, these infections were almost unknown.

'Sell by' and 'use by' dates are a brilliant invention of food manufacturers to legitimize the wasting of huge quantities of perfectly usable food. Which of us would not know if the food we supplied to our family had seriously gone off? In most cases this would be long after the 'sell-by' date. The reality is that most food poisoning comes from quite specific bacteria which would be beyond detection even by the most vigilant among us, as the food will usually appear quite normal.

Obviously, babies are very susceptible to infections until they have had a chance to develop some immunities, so a high level of sterility is important, particularly with the equipment used for feeding them. This is one of the many advantages of breastfeeding, which not only supplies young babies with antibodies in the breast milk, but is also naturally sterile.

Please Note

My comments about excessive efforts to avoid contact with bacteria should not be taken to mean that personal hygiene is not important. Infections and infestations in the faeces can be passed to other humans and, being specialized invaders, can have very unpleasant effects. Washing hands after going to the lavatory and before preparing food is of paramount importance.

DORMANT TROUBLE

Many children have very strong lymphatic systems and, despite modern conditions, are remarkably resistant and resilient to illness in their early years. By the age of seven or eight, they have a wide range of circulating antibodies and are able to fight common infections without any obvious difficulty. However, the lymphatic systems of a fair proportion of others are not so robust – either as a result of their genes, the impact of an acute infection such as a serious strep throat early in life, or the repercussions of our modern lifestyle. These children have a miserable first few years plagued by a constant stream of sore throats, colds and other infections.

Young children who are constantly unwell may appear to 'grow out' of their susceptibility by around seven years of age – and the early setbacks are all but forgotten as parents breathe a huge sigh of relief. However, in many cases the underlying trouble still remains unresolved and the effects, for example, of damaged tonsils on the child's long-term health may only become apparent later in life. They have simply got to a stage where they have already made antibodies against all the common bacteria and thanks to the combination of their store of immunities and the efficiency of other defence mechanisms within the body, they can tolerate everyday infection.

In these cases the lymphatic system has taken such a battering that it may not fully recover without treatment both to clear the lymph nodes and to stimulate the body's natural defences. By the time these children reach their mid-twenties – when their natural repair mechanism starts to slow down – it is quite common for the problems to start up again, often following an assault by a particularly virulent infection such as influenza.

Josh, 29, came to see me with sinus trouble and bronchitis. He explained that, as a child, he had had a large number of colds and sore throats. These gradually tailed off as he got older and, by the time he was eight years old, his resistance had improved and he was quite well.

When he was 24, he had a bad attack of flu accompanied by sinus trouble and bronchitis. The flu took its course, but he was left with painful sinuses and a tendency to bronchitis. When I saw him he was still catching frequent infections, which went straight to his chest. He had been given various courses of antibiotics, but the trouble always returned.

On examination I felt a number of enlarged, hard lymph nodes in his neck. I deduced that these had become partially blocked by the infections in his youth and that, as soon as he had acquired all his immunities and had the resilience of youth on his side, he had made an apparent recovery. However, the flu had overloaded his still defective defence system and reactivated the problem caused by the blocked lymph nodes.

Treatment with physical medicine to unblock the lymph nodes and restore proper drainage from the sinus, throat and bronchial membranes stopped further attacks.

LYMPHATIC TIME LINE

Birth	Newborn babies have a high quota of mother's antibodies circulating, so the lymphatic system is fairly inactive.
2–3 months	Once babies are exposed to a range of germs, the different components of the lymphatic system – especially the six tonsils – work flat out to manufacture antibodies. They continue at this level for several years.
6–7 years	Children have generally come into contact with all the everyday bacteria they are likely to by now (apart from the odd seasonal 'bug'), so lymphatic activity starts to ease off.
12 years	As the tonsils and adenoids are not needed, they start to shrink.
17–18 years	By late adolescence, the tonsils virtually cease to function and disappear.
Post-adolescence	The general activity of the lymphatic system falls off, in line with the slowing down of the body as a whole, although it remains competent to deal with the majority of infections it comes into contact with.

THE ANTIBIOTICS QUESTION

The use of antibiotics represents one of the most important advances in modern medicine. In my view, they are some of the most valuable drugs in the pharmacopoeia, but, because of their enormous power and effectiveness, they are also some of the most widely abused.

The real value of antibiotics is in relieving a distressing or damaging infection, or one that is a threat to life or future health. As a routine treatment for people with minor infections, antibiotics give extremely unsatisfactory results and only act to weaken the body's own powers of defence and repair.

It is important to understand that viruses are quite different to bacteria and are **not** affected by antibiotics. In fact, an antibiotic given when the infection is a virus will often eliminate bacteria that kept the virus partly under control. Later in a viral infection, bacteria may take advantage of the weakened system and invade, causing a secondary infection which may require antibiotics to bring it under control.

If children are given antibiotics for every infection they catch, their bodies' own defences never really get a chance to develop and they do not form the wide range of antibodies needed to arm themselves against future infections.

I saw Brian when he was 14. He had been a slightly snuffly child and caught colds very readily up to the age of seven. He would then develop a very sore throat and a fairly high temperature, and remain ill for several days. He was given antibiotics but these did not entirely eliminate the infection. A few months later he would have another sore throat and again be given antibiotics. These infections were recurring every six months and his general health was poor. Added to this, he was behaving badly at school and had very limited powers of concentration. The antibiotics became gradually less and less effective, the attacks more prolonged and his general health slowly deteriorated. Finally his parents became desperate and brought him to see me.

On examination he had very large and unhealthy-looking tonsils, huge lymph nodes and a chain of smaller nodes leading down to his collarbone. I arranged to have his tonsils taken out; one of which turned out to have an abscess in it. His health improved greatly after the operation, although he still had the occasional mild sore throat. I gave him some treatment with ultrasonic waves, massaged his lymph nodes and, after five visits or so, the lymph nodes had virtually gone back to their normal size. The infections gradually became less frequent and after about a year he was extremely fit. At school, his concentration and performance improved enormously.

Another patient, Peter, aged eight, was referred to me because he was having problems with his ears. His doctor, who was known to give antibiotics only very rarely, wondered if the enlarged lymph nodes might mean trouble later in his life.

Peter had had a sore throat some years before, but recovered without the use of antibiotics in about five days and remained well for six years before he went down with this ear infection. Peter obviously had a strong lymphatic system and, as the enlarged lymph nodes were soft, I thought it more than likely that he would get over the infection by himself and that his ears would settle down. In fact the lymph nodes returned to normal without any treatment and Peter remained fit and well.

A research study reported in the medical journals compared two groups of a thousand children of a similar age who were suffering from similar types of sore throat. One group was treated with antibiotics, the other was not.

The average duration of sore throats among the children who were not treated with antibiotics was four days. The recurrence rate was three per cent over the following five years.

The children who were treated with antibiotics took an average of three days to recover, but had a recurrence rate of 68 per cent.

This suggests that antibiotics should not be the first choice of treatment for sore throats and should be reserved instead for when the infection is serious and accompanied by a high temperature, when the ear is involved or when some other complication occurs that needs to be dealt with quickly.

One of the problems with the use of antibiotics is the misconception about what constitutes a 'course' of the drug. A patient who is given enough tablets for five or seven days is often satisfied that this is the correct amount to cure their immediate problem – even worse, the doctor tells them that this is the course for their infection – even though they are not free of the trouble by the end of that time.

Antibiotics act as an anaesthetic on the bacteria, slowing them down to give the body an opportunity to mop up. Depending on the virulence or toughness of the bacteria and their susceptibility to the antibiotic, they will succumb more or less readily to the effects of the drug.

The bacteria within a single colony will have widely varying powers of resistance. This means that, in the early days of taking antibiotics, the sufferer overcomes the very weakest, followed by the weak, later still the mild and, finally, the strongest strains of the bacteria. It follows, therefore, that if an antibiotic is abandoned before it has entirely eliminated the infection, the sufferer will be left with the bacteria that pose the biggest threat.

When the antibiotic is stopped, those bacteria that remain begin to multiply, replacing the ones that were killed off, so the new infection consists of the most virulent strain – which is also, of course, much more resistant to the antibiotic.

A course of antibiotics is therefore whatever is needed to eliminate the infection. It might require five days, three weeks or, in rare cases, even a year or more. It should also be given in the strongest safe dosage to knock out the most resistant bacteria as rapidly and completely as possible.

I saw Alice when she was 16 years old. She had started getting sore throats around the age of three and, on each occasion, was given a fixed dose of antibiotics which did not quite clear the infection. The infections became more frequent and she eventually had her tonsils taken out at the age of 10. After this, she was enormously better, although she remained susceptible.

When she came to see me, she was beginning to have ear trouble and also had a moderately severe throat infection. I treated the lymph nodes and put her onto a four-week course of antibiotics. When she stopped taking them the infection began to return, so I immediately continued the antibiotics for another three weeks, which seemed to do the trick. She did have an infection about three months later, but from then on was largely well and as fit as any other person of her age.

Alice's experience highlights the fact that there is no set dose of antibiotics – *each patient needs whatever is the right amount to clear the infection completely and should continue to take them until this has been achieved.*

BASIC GUIDELINES

A doctor will generally prescribe a course of antibiotics based on a reasonable estimate of how long he or she thinks it will take to get on top of an infection. Ideally, the doctor should ask to see you again before the course has run out, so that a decision can be made regarding whether it needs to be extended. Judging by your initial response, the doctor will be in a position to make an informed calculation about how much longer it may now take. He or she should then review the situation at the end of the further extension in case the dosage has proved inadequate.

The correct antibiotic for a given infection should be lethal to the bacteria involved but have little or no effect on the patient. Any adverse effects, such as an allergic reaction or an excessive destruction of the 'friendly' bacteria in the body, tend to occur during the first few days. So long as these are not severe, keeping a patient on most antibiotics for an extended period is a completely safe practice.

Unlike the antibodies that our bodies produce, antibiotics cannot be programmed to eliminate the undesirable bacteria alone. They work on a number of other vulnerable groups, which can include some of the essential bacteria in the body, especially in the bowel. Many people when taking antibiotics become deficient in vitamin B and some of the natural bacterial flora, which may lead to tiredness, depression or inflammation of the bowel.

Normally these bacteria compete with the fungal inhabitants of the gut for food. If the bacteria are removed, then there is considerably more nourishment available for a fungal infection, such as candida, which may then multiply sufficiently to cause symptoms. It is widely thought that taking vitamin B along with antibiotics helps to prevent this. The re-introduction of bacteria by swallowing acidophilus tablets and eating live, natural yoghourt may also be helpful in restoring health during or after a course of antibiotics.

THE DIETARY MINEFIELD

Food sensitivities come about because of the natural reaction of an inflamed stomach to foods it finds particularly hard to deal with. In order to minimize any additional aggravation, the body instantly releases a huge quantity of an anti-inflammatory substance called cortisol. However, the cortisol is soon used up, causing levels to dip to well below normal which, in turn, triggers an increased volume of blood in the capillaries and of various secretions – especially in the bronchial tree and the sinuses – intensifying any existing catarrhal condition.

There are approved skin tests to establish food sensitivities, but the snag with almost all of these is that they relate only to the actual tissue tested. They are, therefore, of little value in telling you what your intestines react to. Blood tests are very accurate but extremely expensive, and if so much as one food substance to which there is a sensitivity is left out – which is easily done – the whole test becomes useless.

A variety of other less scientific methods are employed for assessing food sensitivities, but I am doubtful as to their effectiveness. My advice to people is to have a blood test performed or use an elimination diet.

LISTEN TO YOUR BODY

You can usually tell if you are particularly sensitive to a food, either because you don't like it (in which case you try to avoid it) or, much more commonly, because you are excessively keen on it. When the food sensitivity is well developed, as soon as you take that particular food into your system your body counteracts the effect of it with a huge surge of cortisone from the adrenal gland. This gives you a feeling of immense well-being, which you come to associate with that food. As the effect of the cortisone dies off, a feeling of lowness and depression sets in and your subconscious immediately craves more of the offending food to give you a further lift.

There are some foods which upset the digestive systems of a fairly high percentage of the population. Wheat and dairy products both fall into this category. Every effort should be made to find alternatives whenever possible. The following suggestions may be useful.

Wheat Alternatives

- Rice – grains, cakes, noodles, breakfast cereals
- Potatoes – baked/boiled/mashed, etc., potato cakes and snacks, potato flour
- Oats – porridge, breakfast cereals, oatcakes, flapjacks
- Corn – cornflakes, polenta, sweetcorn, corn chips, tortillas, popcorn, cornflour
- Rye – pure rye bread and crispbread
- Buckwheat – pasta and pancakes

Dairy Alternatives

- Non-dairy margarine
- Goat's milk/cheese/yoghourt
- Sheep's milk/cheese/yoghourt
- Soya milk and yoghourt: tofu
- Mayonnaise
- Oils – olive, sunflower, sesame, groundnut, walnut, hazelnut, etc. Remember, however, that a few people can be extremely allergic to some nuts
- Hummous; pastes made of olives/peppers/aubergines, etc. for spreading

Breastfeeding your child, if possible, can circumvent a lot of problems in the early years. All too often cow's milk is given as a substitute for breast milk, but our digestive systems do not always tolerate it well. Personally, I think cow's milk should carry a government health warning. Milk is so widely considered to be an essential ingredient of a wholesome diet that many parents worry if their children do not like it. There is no need. Children have a remarkable ability to choose the foods that their bodies need, except where sugar is involved.

This point is clearly illustrated by a 10-year experiment carried out in the United States some years ago. It involved 9,000 orphan children in institutions, between the ages of one and seven, who were divided into three groups.

The first group was fed on a diet which had been specially devised by top dietitians and paediatricians.

The second group was fed on whatever diet they normally had.

The third group was allowed to eat exactly what they wanted from a selection of everyday foods. They could eat as much as they wanted of whatever kind of food they liked whenever they chose, and if they wanted something specific it was given to them. There was no control over their intake, except that sugar was excluded from their diet.

The results showed little difference between the first and second groups, but the third group stood out as being by far the most healthy. This was backed up by x-ray evidence which revealed a marked increase in the growth and density of the bones among the children in the self-regulating group.

When researchers tried to analyse the diet of this group, there was one overwhelming conclusion – that no analysis was possible. The eating habits of each child followed a different pattern, and all were subject to fads that frequently changed. Some ate only one thing, some restricted their intake to just a few foods, while others happily consumed many different foods. The only common strand was the lack of interest in milk, which, given their impressive bone growth, confirms that it is not essential to a healthy diet.

Left to their own devices, then, children will eat what they need when they need it. The glaring exception to this rule is sugar. Perhaps because it is the perfect form of fuel for the body in small quantities

– the body converts all our food into sugar for energy – we find it difficult to exercise our powers of discrimination and self-control when it comes to consuming sweet things! Sugar is an acquired taste which often develops at a young age when adults start giving children sweets and other sugary foods. Once you develop a 'sweet tooth', it is very hard to lose it.

Sugar is also the ideal fuel for bacteria and yeasts (fungi). Eating sweet foods encourages all the bacteria present in your body to multiply. An excess of sugar in the diet also upsets the sugar/fat metabolism, which can cause a number of problems including hardening of the arteries. The connection between sugar consumption and tooth decay is an accepted fact.

DIETARY SUPPLEMENTS

Most of the patients who come to see me need extra vitamins and minerals. The accepted view used to be that our requirements of these substances could be completely met by our dietary intake and that it was unnecessary – probably even harmful – to supplement them. However, more recent research has shown that many people have deficiencies of one sort or another and can benefit from taking the right dietary supplements.

Even though your diet may contain all the nutrients you need, you cannot assume that your body will absorb all the nutrients you take in. In some cases your body may destroy them or use them up faster than is good for you; in others, it may not absorb them properly.

For example, if you are suffering from gastritis it can affect the absorption of vitamin B, magnesium and other trace substances. Anxiety states, infection and depression often result in a massive destruction of vitamin B and the excretion of magnesium; associated absorption problems may mean the body is not able to replace these nutrients readily.

The vitamins which usually need to be supplemented are A, B and C. I believe that children and adults should take the recommended daily doses (RDA) of cod liver oil capsules to ensure adequate vitamin A. It is also important for children to have extra vitamin B (best taken in liquid form) throughout their growing lives. Adults, particularly over the age of 45, should choose synthetic formulations of vitamin B, as natural sources often contain yeast and sometimes phytic acid, which can upset the digestive system. Magnesium, which tends to be excreted when a person is under stress, is needed to make the red cells in the blood work.

RDA	CHILDREN (UNDER 12)	ADULTS
Vitamin A	pro rata by weight	800 µg (not if pregnant or planning to become pregnant)
Vitamin B	pro rata by weight	B complex up to 1 g a day as directed
Vitamin C	500 mg (50–250 mg for children under 4)	1–2 gm (3–4 gm following infection or injury)
Cod liver oil	strengths vary, follow instructions on the bottle	not to be taken if pregnant
Acidophilus tablet (with/following antibiotic)		as per instructions
Potassium citrate (cystitis)		as per instructions
Magnesium	100–200 mg/day	Magnesium OK is a good product which includes other trace elements

Even if you eat plenty of fresh fruit and vegetables you cannot be sure you are getting enough vitamin C, as levels are often depleted in artificially ripened produce. It is almost impossible to take too much vitamin C, as excessive quantities can cause diarrhoea – your body's way of telling you to take a bit less! However, reducing the dosage after a prolonged period of high doses (1 g or more a day) may result in scurvy.

If your child finds it hard to take a vitamin tablet and it is not available in fluid form, an effective method is to crush it to a powder and use a syringe to blow it into her mouth, where it will then dissolve. Alternatively, get your child to fill her mouth with water and then put the tablets in – they will both be swallowed together.

Many people are lacking in essential minerals and benefit considerably from taking a mineral supplement. However, caution is the watchword here. When I asked a patient recently if she took any extra vitamins or minerals, she put 27 bottles on my table, each one labelled for a particular purpose: relieving painful periods, enhancing skin, preventing colds and so on. Each bottle contained much the same minerals and, as a result, she was taking a fairly serious overdose, spending a great deal of money and solving nothing.

Minerals, also known as trace elements, are nearly all metals or metalloids which, if taken in excess, are toxic to the body. For this reason the body has an in-built mechanism to prevent you from absorbing too much of any one. However, your body does not distinguish between each individual substance, but reacts to them *en masse*. When a critical level is reached, the body will block any further absorption, which means that by taking too much of one mineral you may be missing out on all the other essential trace elements.

I would recommend taking one supplement which contains all the necessary trace elements. The only exception is zinc, which is probably best taken separately, perhaps at night, as it tends to react with the others and then may not be absorbed.

A CLOSER LOOK AT LYMPHATIC STRUCTURES AND NODES

5

THE TONSILS, ADENOIDS AND APPENDIX

Everybody knows that things can go wrong with your tonsils and appendix and, if the problem gets serious, you may end up having them removed; but how many people know the critical role which these parts of our anatomy play in our body's defence system?

When it comes to fighting infection in the throat and bowel, the tonsils, adenoids and appendix are in the front line of defence – the first protective mechanisms to be activated. If the walls of these strongholds are attacked and broken down, this can cause a series of related – and yet quite separate – problems.

In order to provide strong protection against possible assault by bacteria, the human body has a disproportionately large amount of lymphoid tissue in the mouth and throat area. This includes the (fancial) tonsils, lingual tonsils and adenoids, and numerous other lymph deposits scattered all over the area (see page 63).

THE TONSILS

Your tonsils are under continuous siege from bacteria in the mouth that have been either breathed in or carried in on food, as well as from bacteria that come down from the nose. We know that healthy tonsils are capable of overcoming a wide variety of infections.

However, a point may be reached where the tonsils – especially if they are inherently weak or have been weakened by previous damage – can no longer cope. This is usually for one of the following reasons:

■ their channels have become blocked by the accumulation of debris and damage from a number of separate infections

■ they have been overwhelmed by a single infection from a very powerful bug

---

THE LEGACY OF DAMAGED TONSILS

If damaged tonsils are not removed, they can cause prolonged ill health or serious illness. Although symptoms other than a sore throat may not necessarily be present at an early age, they may arise later in life. All of the following conditions may arise from damaged tonsils: recurrent sore throats, tonsillitis, quinsey, sinusitis, middle ear infections, inflamed joints and kidneys, skin rashes, constant tiredness, poor short-term memory and concentration, an uncooperative attitude.

When healthy tonsils are active in the presence of an infection, the lymph drains from them into the tonsil node, which is just below the angle of the jaw (see diagram on page 63). After repeated infections, the assistance provided by the node will diminish as it fills up with debris. The more obstructed the node becomes, the less effective the drainage, and the greater the load on the tonsils.

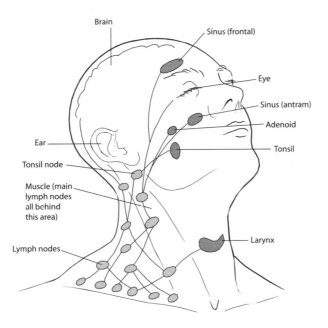

Brain

Sinus (frontal)

Eye

Sinus (antram)

Adenoid

Ear

Tonsil

Tonsil node

Muscle (main lymph nodes all behind this area)

Larynx

Lymph nodes

▲ CERVICAL NODES

Eventually there comes a point when the tonsils can no longer defend themselves adequately against the bacteria attacking from outside, which then invade and damage the structure of the tonsils themselves. At this stage, the blood supply to the damaged tonsils is so reduced that antibiotics have little chance of overcoming these unwelcome invaders either.

The tonsils become, in effect, a comfortable rest home for tired bacteria to recuperate and multiply in preparation for a further attack on the throat – then or at a later date. This sorry state of the individual's defences means that any 'bug' that comes along can take up residence. The longer the situation lasts, the greater the burden on the lymphatic drainage of the throat area. Predictably, the attacks also become increasingly virulent and frequent and harder to shake off.

The solution is not necessarily to give antibiotics at the first sign of a sore throat. People should be encouraged to acquire immunities to the widest possible range of bacteria to reduce the likelihood of succumbing to the same infection again, although, in the case of a 'strep' throat – which is usually accompanied by a fairly high temperature and a general malaise – it is advisable to give an antibiotic at an early stage to avoid permanent damage to the tonsils and their subsequent removal. A simple case of tonsillitis will usually clear up on its own in three or four days.

Tonsillitis means inflammation of the tonsils, and is a sign that their defence mechanism has been activated against an invading bacterium. The classic symptoms are:

- redness
- swelling
- pain
- heat (local, but also a general rise in body temperature)
- loss of function (difficulty in swallowing).

The tonsils are more than a match for a wide range of bacteria and will generally produce antibodies to destroy the invader.

If a child suffers from recurrent sore throats and the tonsils do not seem to be damaged, then attention must be focused on his or her general health. There is plenty that you can do at home. Fresh fruit and vegetables are important. Extra vitamins may be needed – most probably vitamins A and D in the form of cod liver oil or halibut oil, plus vitamin C. Depending on the age and size of the child, up to 1 gm a day of vitamin C can be beneficial (see page 56), gradually cutting down to 200 mg a day as the infection begins to pass.

I would advise plenty of fresh air, reduced heating and the lightest layer of clothing. Massaging the enlarged lymph nodes in the neck (see page 215 in the Treatment section) will usually bring about considerable improvement. This can be carried out at home, although in severe cases it may be advisable to follow up with a visit to a physiotherapist for ultrasonic and electrical treatment to the tonsil and associated lymph nodes.

CONGESTION AND CATARRH

The standard response to infection or irritation in the nose and throat area is for the mucous membranes to swell and increase their secretions in an attempt to wash away the invading bug or irritant. The resulting congestion in the area, almost inevitably compounded as the lymph nodes in the neck start to silt up and overflow, causes the membranes to become waterlogged as this extra fluid now has nowhere to drain. Mucus first appears in the nose and throat, giving rise to a runny nose and cough. It may also drain down the windpipe – especially at night – and infect the breathing tubes, resulting in bronchitis. Once the membranes have become irritated, the conditions are ripe for allergies and asthma to develop (see page 123).

Michael was 15 when he came to see me. He had been a perfectly healthy baby but, by the time he was about two, he had begun to catch a number of colds each year. Gradually he became more and more catarrhal, until he had a runny and blocked nose most of the time and life had become pretty miserable. He then started to go down with one sore throat after another. Eventually, at the age of eight, he had his tonsils and adenoids removed.

Michael's general condition improved a great deal after this operation, but unfortunately he still had a blocked and runny nose and was very susceptible to colds. He had also started to develop sensitivities and seemed to have almost constant hay fever throughout the year. He underwent skin sensitivity tests which showed that he was slightly allergic to a number of different substances. He had been put onto anti-histamine drugs, which dried his nose up for a while, but their effect slowly wore off.

When he came to see me he was a little slow in his academic development, his concentration was patchy and he was rather naughty, with a reputation for being cheeky to the teachers. His short-term memory was poor and he lost his temper easily. On examination, his nose had very swollen membranes and there was some discharge coming from the nose and sinus area, although the tonsil beds were healthy. In his neck there were a number of enlarged, hard lymph nodes which could be felt from behind his ear right down to his collarbone.

I diagnosed that the lymph nodes in his neck had become blocked by the constant infection in his tonsils and that, because of this blockage, the overflow was causing the membranes to swell, which weakened their resistance to new infection. In addition, dusts and pollens were becoming lodged in these sticky, swollen membranes.

Normal membranes are shiny and covered with little hairs that sweep irritating particles off the membrane in a coordinated wave towards the mouth. However, in Michael's case the hairs were engulfed in the swollen membrane and not functioning. Thus the particles landed and he reacted to them.

Michael was given 11 treatments to restore normal function to his lymph nodes, at the end of which his health had greatly improved and he found it much easier to concentrate. I was told later that his work and behaviour improved very considerably at school.

Catarrhal secretions can also run down into the stomach, causing the stomach lining to become inflamed. Children with this condition often have very poor appetites. In extreme cases the secretions may drain through the bowel into the lymph nodes in the abdominal cavity. This may ultimately damage the appendix (see below).

Inflammation of the stomach, known as gastritis, makes the stomach more sensitive to certain foods; food intolerances often develop. One of the common effects of this is a reactive swelling of the membranes of the nose, throat and sinuses, which further increases the catarrh. So gastritis is both caused and perpetuated by a catarrhal condition.

TONSILS AND MENTAL FUNCTION

It comes as a great surprise to most people to discover that damaged tonsils can have an impact on mental function and behaviour. The reason for this is that the tonsil nodes are part of a group of lymph nodes in the neck which also drain the brain. If the tonsil nodes become clogged with debris, this can affect drainage from other areas that share the same drainage route – in this case, the brain. This cerebral oedema, as it is called, has the same sort of symptoms as a very mild form of concussion.

Typical sufferers are children who do poorly at school and find it hard to mix with others. Teachers may criticize them for lack of concentration, poor short-term memory and irritability. Parents find that these children are very often tired and object strongly to being told what to do. Children who experience these difficulties arouse my sympathy, as they are often punished for behaviour which they find impossible to control. It is remarkable how a child's personality can be transformed once the damaged tonsils are removed and proper drainage from the brain is restored.

Adults are equally liable to experience these effects as a result of blocked tonsil nodes. The difference is that the changes are usually less conspicuous because their behaviour and performance are not monitored in the same way as a child's and they are better at compensating for any malfunction.

I was at a dinner party some years ago when another guest enquired when the school holidays started. Overhearing this, our hostess burst into tears and fled from the room. Her husband signalled to me urgently to follow her, so I went out and asked her what was wrong. She replied that she was dreading her son Christopher's return from school. She said that he was a truly ghastly child – difficult, rude and obnoxious. Apparently Christopher, who was only nine years of age, was making her life utterly miserable and she hated the holidays.

I was really taken aback at this outburst, because I had known Christopher for several years and he had always struck me as a very pleasant and polite boy. I asked a lot of questions and it emerged that he had been a very easy child up until the age of five, when he had a bad attack of flu, followed by sore throats and tonsil trouble. Soon after, he had another attack of flu and, from then on, he was constantly afflicted with sore throats and seemed very prone to infection. At about the age of seven, Christopher started becoming very difficult and uncooperative. His family believed this change in behaviour was due to the fact that he had gone to boarding school too early and felt rejected.

I was not so sure that the problem was psychological, so I asked her to bring Christopher to see me during the school holidays. On examination, he had some nasty-looking, infected tonsils and it looked as though he had had a number of infections in his ears. I also noted some enlarged tonsil lymph nodes and a chain of swollen glands leading down from them. I suggested that the behavioural problem might stem from cerebral congestion and that his tonsils should be removed.

After this was done, Christopher came to have a few treatments to clear his lymph nodes. Within a few weeks he had reverted to his former helpful and willing self – and school holidays were no longer a nightmare for his mother.

If a child displays this kind of behavioural pattern, or has an obvious change in personality, then there may be a number of physical causes. Underlying disorders such as a cerebral tumour or food sensitivities are more likely to be diagnosed, but catarrhal problems should not be ruled out as a possible cause. It is astonishing what a difference treatment can make and how this can alter the course of a child's future life and development. I feel very strongly that teachers and parents should be made aware of this extremely common and unacknowledged cause of bad behaviour.

REMOVAL OF TONSILS

I cannot emphasize too strongly that, if tonsils are infected and pouring toxins into the whole body, they should be removed.

Parents frequently say they have been told that their children's tonsils, although damaged, should be left in. If your child has recurrent sore throats and seems to catch a lot of colds then you should question why. Suggest to your doctor that your child has his tonsils taken out. If he disagrees, but you feel strongly that this is the best course of action, then insist that it is done. Do not be fobbed off with comments such as 'he'll grow out of it'. The symptoms may subside, but this does not mean that the lymphatic system is in full working order.

There is rarely a penalty for removing healthy tonsils, as other lymphoid tissue will take over their functions if required, whereas the consequences of leaving infected tonsils in – apart from immediate ill-health – can be very serious. I see a number of patients every year in middle age who are suffering from arthritis, tiredness, ME and other problems which could have been avoided if their tonsils had been removed at an early age.

It is vital to distinguish between enlarged tonsils, which may be working hard and successfully to ward off infection, and damaged tonsils, which are a health hazard and must be removed. Similar confusion can surround the fate of a damaged appendix, which, if it is not removed, can cause serious and prolonged ill-health.

If in doubt, the following guidelines may be helpful. Tonsils should be removed if they appear small and pale or if they are large and infected *and* the patient shows some of these clinical signs:

- the tonsil lymph node (located under the angle of the jaw) feels enlarged, firm or hard, and is permanently tender, i.e. painful in response to pressure
- there is a history of frequent sore throats and a tendency to catch lingering colds
- there is evidence of irritability, poor short-term memory, tiredness, lack of concentration and poor performance at school or work.

The tonsils are self-contained units in a capsule, joined to the body by a stalk containing the artery, veins, lymphatic ducts and connective tissue (see diagram). If the tonsil is removed in childhood then it is a fairly simple operation – severing the stalk will enable the tonsil to be slipped out of its capsule quite cleanly. The stalk may then need tying off, or may just seal itself off. This is a very minor operation causing the minimum of disturbance to the patient.

If, however, destroyed or damaged tonsils are left in place for a number of years, the patient will, at the very least, suffer sore throats, constant infections and excessive tiredness and may develop more serious

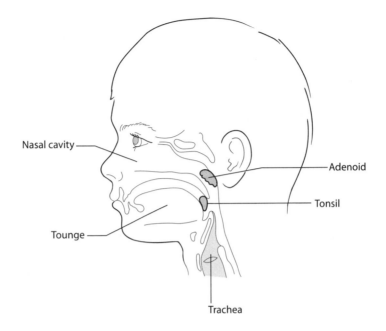

Nasal cavity

Adenoid

Tonsil

Tounge

Trachea

health problems. A further danger associated with infected tonsils is that, once the inflammation reaches the outer edge of the organ, it will cause the capsule itself to become inflamed and sticky so that the tonsils adhere to the throat. Blood vessels then grow across this gap and the tonsils slowly become merged with the surrounding tissues.

If the tonsils then become troublesome and need to be removed at a later date, the operation is an altogether more formidable undertaking. The tonsils have to be cut out of the throat wall, leaving a large raw area and the possibility of incomplete removal since there is no clear definition between the tonsils and the throat. This can jeopardize the outcome of the operation, and may require further surgery in the future.

Post-operative recovery is obviously far less smooth than if the tonsils can be removed from an intact capsule. After about the tenth day, bacteria tend to settle in the raw area where the tonsils were cut away, causing a similar infection to that in the original tonsils. It is not until the normal protective throat membrane has grown over the whole area, about two months later, that the bacteria are finally thrown out, with all the expected benefits and improvements in the condition of the throat itself and the general health of the patient.

A CASE OF MISTAKEN IDENTITY

It is not unusual for the adenoids to be removed instead of the tonsils due to a misunderstanding about their role and function. Ear, nose and throat specialists tend to focus on the size of the structures, and seldom consider the lymph nodes as a critical aid to diagnosis. When the tonsils are no longer effectively repelling and resisting infection, the adenoids increase in size because they are forced to take on some of the tonsils' workload. For this reason, it is the healthy adenoids – and not the diseased tonsils – that are often the subject of the surgeon's knife.

Adrian, 14, was very catarrhal and congested and had a tendency to breathe through his mouth. He said that he felt unwell, got tired easily and had poor concentration, which was backed up by bad school reports. At the age of nine he had had his adenoids taken out because of the respiratory obstruction. As the nasal passage around the adenoids is rather narrow, breathing can be impeded if they become considerably enlarged. However, this had helped his breathing only for a short time. Subsequently his overall condition seemed to deteriorate.

When I examined him I found that his throat was red and he had large, unhealthy-looking tonsils. The tonsil lymph nodes were very swollen and tender and there was also a chain of enlarged lymph nodes leading down either side of his neck. This picture indicated that the tonsils were damaged and permanently infected and that the other lymph nodes in the area were carrying the extra load.

It transpired that his adenoids had been removed in error, leaving him more vulnerable to infection than ever. Had his tonsils been taken out and his adenoids left in, they would almost certainly have shrunk back to a normal size once they did not have to cope with the stream of infection from the tonsils. He would then have been left with a high resistance to infection and properly functioning lymph nodes.

Adrian had treatment to the lymph nodes in his neck on seven occasions to clear the now significant blockage which had resulted from all the tonsil infections. After that, he felt very fit and has remained so.

The worst thing you can do is to remove healthy adenoids and leave in heavily infected tonsils, which will continue to do damage. The best course is to remove the tonsils and for the surgeon carefully to assess at the time of the operation whether it is necessary to remove the adenoids as well. Thankfully, as already mentioned, the lymph system is so versatile that, if the body should find itself with neither, it will grow new lymph tissue to take the place of the tonsils. **Adenoids should almost never be removed on their own**.

THE APPENDIX

In the same way that the tonsils are the first line of defence against infections of the nose and throat, the appendix provides protection for the bowel wall.

The lymphatic system in the bowel is normally extremely powerful. If the appendix is overloaded, however, then the abdominal lymph nodes – into which it drains – may become congested with the resulting debris and fail to do their job, causing the appendix to become inflamed and infected.

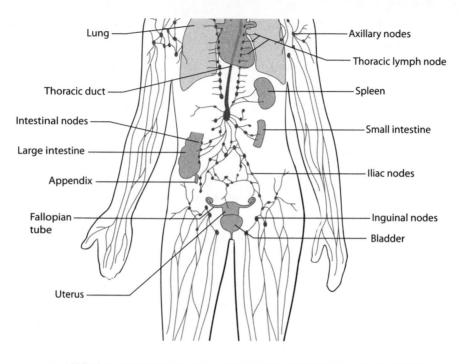

Lung

Axillary nodes

Thoracic lymph node

Thoracic duct

Spleen

Intestinal nodes

Small intestine

Large intestine

Appendix

Iliac nodes

Fallopian
tube

Inguinal nodes

Bladder

Uterus

▲ APPENDIX, PERITONEUM AND ASSOCIATED ABDOMINAL LYMPH NODES

Low-grade infections in the walls of the appendix are initially controlled by the antibody response and the fighting white cells, and there may well be no obvious symptoms. However, each attack leaves more scarring in the wall of the appendix, usually halfway along the tube, which progressively and then permanently narrows the channel.

The membrane lining the appendix secretes mucus as part of its defence mechanism, but the membrane also swells and, in extreme cases, the combination of the scarring and the swelling may narrow the opening to such a point that it becomes almost completely blocked and there is nowhere for the mucus to go.

As the obstruction increases, foreign material is more likely to become trapped in the appendix. Just as damaged tonsils become a home for bacteria to live in and attack as they please, so the appendix serves as a perfect culture medium for infections from the bowel. In some cases, the appendix may perforate and form a local abscess or release pus into the abdominal cavity. This results in a very serious condition known as peritonitis, which was often fatal in the days before modern treatment with antibiotics.

CHRONIC APPENDICITIS

Unfortunately, the early signs of a troubled appendix are often missed and the condition can continue for some time – sometimes over several years – causing much distress. Often it is not diagnosed until it is too late and the condition has developed into acute appendicitis. Occasionally there are no symptoms associated with chronic appendicitis (sometimes referred to as a 'grumbling appendix') but here are some warning signs to look out for.

- Pain about two inches above the navel is felt in the early stages when there is a low-grade inflammation in the appendix wall.
- If the infection breaks through the appendix and inflames the peritoneum lining the outside of the appendix, then the pain switches to the actual site and is felt in the lower right side of the abdomen.
- If the tummy ache suddenly turns into a much sharper pain in the right side of the stomach, this means that the infection is breaking through to the peritoneum and the patient should be taken to hospital immediately.

ASSOCIATED PAINS IN THE BLADDER

Problems with the appendix may also result in pain felt in unexpected places such as the back or bladder or even in the knee. Women in particular often present with an irritable bladder, passing urine frequently and complaining about a condition that feels like cystitis. These symptoms arise because the inflamed appendix touches these parts of the body and also affects nearby nerves, producing 'referred pain' elsewhere in the body. Due to the nature of the nerve system, the pain resulting from an inflamed nerve is felt at the place the nerve actually supplies, not at the site of its stimulation.

GENERAL ILL-HEALTH

Children, or indeed adults, with chronic appendicitis are generally unwell. Characteristic symptoms include:

- continual tiredness and/or episodes of exhaustion for no apparent reason
- poor appetite
- alternating constipation and diarrhoea.

In addition, there may be sub-acute attacks of appendicitis with characteristic stomach pains accompanied by:

- nausea
- greyness in the face and a tell-tale waxy white ring around the mouth
- a feeling of being threatened, with a tendency to burst into tears.

These symptoms are often diagnosed as a condition known as abdominal adenitis, because it is thought they are caused by inflamed abdominal lymph nodes. I have always found this assumption rather unsatisfactory, as lymph nodes are inert objects and they don't become inflamed by themselves – something inflames them. A common scenario is that pus from the tonsils is swallowed, upsetting the bowel and appendix. The symptoms of 'abdominal adenitis' are almost always cured by taking out the appendix.

A child may suffer from chronic appendicitis with sub-acute attacks for several years. Despite the fact that the child is obviously not thriving, a parent is often told that the symptoms will pass. The symptoms may indeed subside a little, but the appendix remains like a time-bomb waiting to explode. When you feel the stomach of someone with a damaged appendix, the muscles in the lower right hand side of the abdomen will be tight. This condition, known as muscle guarding, is nature's way of making a wall to protect the delicate appendix from the outside and is one of the classic signs that all is not well. When the appendix is removed under these conditions, it is usually found to be infected. Pressure on this area causes pain from the inflamed appendix.

If a damaged appendix is left in it can take something as small as a change of food on holiday or an attack of enteritis to trigger acute appendicitis. The earlier a damaged appendix is diagnosed, the sooner it can be removed – avoiding a serious health risk.

The main causes of damage to the appendix are:

- low-grade throat infections early in life
- poor diet, especially too little roughage
- excessive amounts of laxatives, spicy or 'sensitizing' foods.

EARLY THROAT INFECTIONS

As we have seen, when children are subject to many throat infections, the tonsils may simply be unable to cope. Phlegm and pus packed with bacteria drain down from the tonsils to the stomach, bowel and possibly even the appendix. This additional infection can prove too much for an already overworked appendix and it becomes unable to defend itself against attack.

Clara was 17 when she was brought to see me. She had had problems with her throat since she was about seven years of age, consisting of two or three sore throats a year. From the age of about 12 she found that she became tired easily and was not concentrating very well at school. She had also lost her appetite and become a faddy eater. She complained at times of vague pains in her tummy just above the navel.

On examination I found that Clara had large and heavily infected tonsils as well as enlarged, tender tonsil nodes. There was also a degree of tightening of the muscles in the lower right part of her abdomen, where the appendix lies. This area was very tender to the touch.

My first action was to get Clara's tonsils removed, as these were most likely to be causing a problem. After this, her general health improved. However, she still tired very easily, and used to turn very pale and develop a white ring around her mouth. She also continued to suffer from pains in her tummy.

These signs all indicated to me that her appendix had become damaged and that she was having episodes of sub-acute appendicitis.

I consulted a surgeon who agreed to remove her appendix, which was indeed found to be damaged. From then on Clara made a good recovery in every respect.

POOR DIET

A frequent cause of damage to the appendix is a poor diet, especially one that contains too little roughage. This puts the whole bowel under strain.

The bowel moves the food we consume steadily down its length by a ring of muscle contracting so that the passage is almost closed off. This ring moves slowly along the bowel, pushing the food in front of it – similar to the way a caterpillar moves around. If the food mass contains only a small proportion of solids, it does not stimulate the movements of the bowel properly, so proper propulsion of the food does not take place. This can cause irritation, especially of the large bowel.

Camilla, 37, was feeling unwell and had pain in her back, which was particularly acute between the shoulders. These symptoms had been going on intermittently for about 15 years. She also got tired very easily and in the last few years had been having trouble, first of all, with constipation and then an irritable bowel. She ate very little roughage so as not to upset her bowel, but she was finding that she had to take laxatives almost every night if she was to have any motion at all the next day. Her nails were brittle and cracked, she had very dry skin and her hair was thin and dull.

On examination I found that Camilla had an exaggerated curve in her upper back and that her abdomen was tender, especially around the large bowel. The membrane of her throat was red and swollen. Some discharge was also present in her nose. She had a number of enlarged lymph nodes in her neck on both sides and she also had a lot of fluid retention in the muscles at the root of the lung, which tends to indicate that there is trouble in the lymph nodes in that area.

We decided that she had gastritis – probably associated with the back problem – which had caused faulty absorption of vitamin B. This largely accounted for her dry skin, cracked nails, straggly hair and possibly some of her tiredness. It was also clear that her bowel was suffering as a result of the insufficient bulk. So I put her on a high-fibre diet and asked her to try and cut milk out of her diet, as I thought she might have a sensitivity to it.

At first her bowels were very upset, so I put her onto a drug to settle them down for a week or two. Gradually she came off this drug and, after a while, her bowels settled and she began to feel altogether better. She did not need to have her appendix removed as the catarrhal state seemed to have improved dramatically.

As Camilla's story shows, lack of bulk in the diet commonly causes constipation and may also be partly responsible, along with food sensitivities, for an irritable bowel. Other associated problems include: diverticulosis – where little sacs in the bowel wall balloon out, usually at the site of muscle weakness where the blood vessels pass through them – and cancer of the bowel. Although lack of fibre is not the cause of bowel cancer, it is a fact that people who eat a high-fibre diet have a significantly lower incidence of the disease.

While lack of bulk can cause problems with the bowel and adversely affect the appendix, a diet too rich in stimulating substances or foods that loosen the bowel is also to be avoided – as well as any foods to which a person has become sensitive. All of these can hurry food through the system, so that it arrives in the bowel only partly digested.

Bacteria can then infect this semi-fluid food mass, especially if there is already excessive fluid in the area, which makes it much easier for bacteria to spread around the bowel. Toxins from this bacterial activity may also mildly poison the muscles of the bowel wall, causing some degree of constipation. This situation makes the appendix more vulnerable to invasion by bacteria.

6 THE CERVICAL NODES

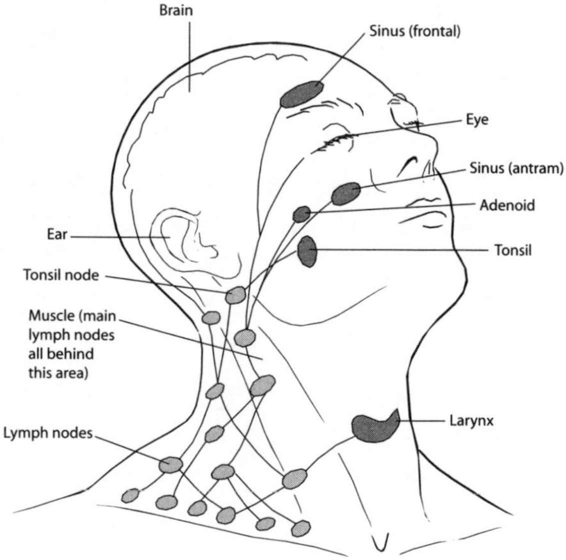

▲ DIAGRAM SHOWING LOCATION OF ALL GROUPS OF CERVICAL NODES + DRAINAGE ROUTES

Labels on diagram:
- Brain
- Sinus (frontal)
- Eye
- Sinus (antram)
- Adenoid
- Tonsil
- Ear
- Tonsil node
- Muscle (main lymph nodes all behind this area)
- Lymph nodes
- Larynx

When a group of lymph nodes silts up with debris, the whole area is undermined by the resulting poor drainage, but usually only one part of the area becomes noticeably affected. There are probably a number of different reasons for this: working in a poorly ventilated, centrally heated environment, for example, could weaken the sinuses and make them the centre of trouble. However, a congenital weakness (such as too small a drainage hole) is a much more common cause of sinus problems.

This increased susceptibility of one area could be compared to a link in a chain with a design fault. The chain, representing all the different tissues in one area, would never break under normal usage. If subjected to unusual stress, however, this weak link would be the one affected.

This section looks at the complications that can arise when the lymph nodes in the head and neck become congested. As the diagram on the previous page shows, the cervical nodes are located in a triangle in the neck formed at the top by the ear and running down to one end of the collarbone in the front and the other end at the back. The upper ones tend to be associated with conditions affecting the sinuses, ears, throat and tonsils, the lower ones with the bronchial tree. A permanently nasal voice, a tendency to breathe through the mouth and a puffy complexion are often external indications of longstanding blockages in these lymph nodes.

In the days before more sophisticated diagnostic equipment, the lowest cervical nodes used to be taken out and examined under a microscope to diagnose some of the diseases of the lung.

The upper and more important set of nodes are far more commonly involved in illness than is generally realized. They can become over-burdened if:

■ they are progressively obstructed by a series of minor throat infections

■ the products of infection from damaged tonsils drain continually into them

■ they are overwhelmed by one acute throat infection.

We already know that, when lymph nodes become overloaded, this leads to back-pressure of fluid in the neighbouring lymphatic vessels, causing:

■ the associated membranes to swell with fluid

■ lowered resistance to infection due to poor circulation of the tissue fluids and resulting thick, unhealthy membranes.

In these conditions a variety of complaints can arise. However, in most cases treatment to improve the drainage eases the problem by relieving the back-pressure and reducing the swelling.

EAR PROBLEMS

Obstruction of the cervical nodes which drain the ears leads to the swelling of various related membranes, causing a range of possible problems.

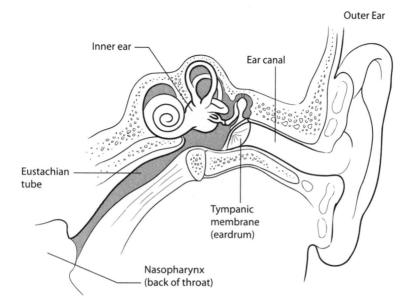

Outer Ear

Inner ear

Ear canal

Eustachian
tube

Tympanic
membrane
(eardrum)

Nasopharynx
(back of throat)

▲ SIMPLE DIAGRAM OF EAR SHOWING PARTS MENTIONED BELOW

THE OUTER EAR

The outer ear gathers the sound waves and, although some of us can wiggle our ears as a party piece, we are unable to adjust them to an optimum listening position in the way that animals such as dogs can. As sound travels down the 'trumpet' of our outer ear, it is amplified. It then vibrates the ear drum, a membrane that separates the outer ear from the middle ear, and transmits the sound to it. Although sometimes prone to infections and eczema, the outer ear has problems that are usually easily treated by simple measures, so it falls outside the scope of this book.

THE MIDDLE EAR

The sole purpose of the middle ear is to amplify sound, which is achieved by a system of 'leverage' of its three minute ossicles, or bones. The Eustachian tube is a small passage which runs from the middle ear to the back of the throat, emerging near the tonsil. It carries out the all-important function of equalizing the pressure between the air inside and outside the ear. This is essential, as unequal pressures – such as occur with atmospheric changes or when you go up or down in an aeroplane – disturb your eardrum and can cause agonizing pain or even deafness.

THE INNER EAR

The inner ear consists of three completely separate pieces of equipment, each with totally different functions. Although it is one continuous piece of apparatus, it is another example of how parts of our bodies have evolved to perform multiple functions to make room for so much machinery in such a small space.

The inner ear is full of fluid which is in contact with the inner drum and is vibrated by it. The vibrating fluid transmits the sound to the first piece of apparatus, a structure called the *cochlea*, which resembles a snail shell. The cochlea detects the different frequencies in the sound complex and transfers them to nerves that go to the hearing centre in the brain, so this is the part that 'hears'.

The same fluid is used to aid our postural mechanism via the three semi-circular *canals* located in the inner ear. If you turn one of these canals round on its own axis the fluid will remain stationary; in the same way that, if you have a cup of tea with a tea leaf floating on the top, you will find that if you turn the cup round the tea will not turn with it and the tea leaf will stay where it was and not move with the cup. Sensitive hairs in bulges in the canals detect the movement of this fluid and, by combining the information from all six canals in both ears – all on completely different planes – the brain receives very accurate information concerning the movements of your head and body.

The third piece of equipment is a box – the *vestibule* – which contains a number of little stones which fall to the bottom when you are standing upright. As soon as you tilt your head these stones move around and sensors in the tiny hairs throughout the walls of the vestibule detect your position and tell the brain. This means that even if you were in a darkened room or on a moving surface you would have a very accurate assessment of your exact position – however slow or slight the movement.

AIR PRESSURE IMBALANCES

If the Eustachian tube is obstructed, there are two main consequences:

1 air passes less freely through the tube to restore the pressure that accompanies atmospheric changes
2 a vacuum may result.

Blood is designed to absorb gases from the lungs and tissues. There is sufficient blood circulation in the walls of the middle ear to remove a significant quantity of the air present there. If these gases are not replaced by air passing through the Eustachian tube, a vacuum will result. Such a situation, as Sophie's story below shows, can cause severe earache, which may intensify when there is a significant shift in air pressure.

From the age of five, Sophie – who was 11 when she came to see me – used to get earache every time she caught a cold. The pain became more intense and prolonged on each occasion. She was also very catarrhal and had begun to get hay fever in the summer months. She had been on holiday about two months before I saw her and told me how, when the aeroplane took off, she experienced agonizing earache which continued for half an hour. Then there was a loud 'plop' in her ear and the pain suddenly stopped.

On landing she had bad earache again and, for about three hours afterwards, was completely deaf. Then, after a series of gurgles in her ear, the pain gradually went. She was given some antihistamine tablets by a doctor where she was on holiday and, although she had some earache on the return journey, it was not so severe.

When I saw Sophie, her eardrums, particularly the left one, were very retracted and the membranes in her throat were somewhat swollen. She had moderate-sized tonsils and there were large, hard lymph nodes on both sides of her neck. I concluded that the lymph nodes were obstructing the drainage of lymph and that the membranes lining the Eustachian tube were swollen.

This swelling was partially blocking the tube and so stopping the air pressure in the middle ear from equalizing with the outside air. A dramatic change of pressure caused the drum to be drawn across or blown out, resulting in acute earache and deafness. Sophie had nine treatments to the lymph nodes which improved her condition significantly. She did have to come for occasional treatment over the following two years but, after that, the trouble cleared completely.

For more about ear conditions, see the A–Z section.

EYE PROBLEMS

The eye is a unique organ in the body. Since light has to pass from the lens through to the back of the eye without obstruction, there is a cavity behind the pupil of the eye filled with a completely transparent jelly, called *vitreous humour*.

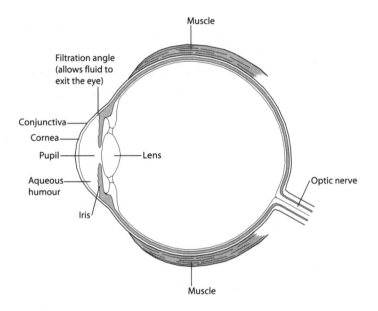

▲ DIAGRAMS OF THE EYE SHOWING PARTS MENTIONED BELOW

The eye is a very remarkable piece of equipment which, in many ways, resembles a camera. The difference is that a camera is a rigid box except for those parts that have to move to allow for focusing. The eye, by contrast, is a soft, elastic ball with the lens situated in a hole in the front (the pupil) and the retina (the equivalent of the film) lining a large section of the circular back of the eyeball.

The vitreous humour is living material and therefore needs its blood supply and drainage, like all other tissues. If, however, it had a network comparable to the rest of the body, there would be little space left for the light. To get round this problem, the various components of the eye depend to a large extent on filtration: fluid filters through the eye and then goes out through little ducts, the drains positioned around the iris (see diagram on page 89).

This works very well in ideal conditions, but since the cells are at the outer limit of distance from the nearest blood vessel, the circulation to them is easily disrupted. Equally, the smallest blockage of the drainage system can have a significant impact on structures in the eye.

The eyeball is designed to revolve in its socket to avoid unnecessary head movements, so there is a gap between the eye and the socket. To prevent dust, foreign bodies or bacteria getting in behind the eye, a loose, transparent membrane called the *conjunctiva* forms a continuous surface on the front of the eye, sealing off the back of the eye and lining the inside of the eyelids and the white of the eye.

Like all mucous membranes, the conjunctiva needs constant lubrication to keep it moist and healthy. This is generated by tear glands in the lids of each eye, which produce a fluid rich in salts and armed with an anti-bacterial substance to ward off infection. The most obvious of its protective roles is to release large quantities of fluid (tears) to wash away any foreign bodies. When the eye membrane becomes infected, the fluid becomes thick and sticky and tends to fasten the eyelids together. This is to prevent further infection entering the eye and also to give the eye a rest, which helps in overcoming the infection.

In order to prevent this constant stream of lubricating fluid from overflowing and running down our cheeks, nature has created a drainage outlet in the form of a large tear duct, the entrance to which can be seen as a tiny pimple at the inner corner of each eye. This duct runs downwards and inwards and passes into your nose (which explains the runny nose that often follows an outburst of tears), eventually draining backwards into your throat.

INGUINAL, ABDOMINAL AND THORACIC LYMPH NODES

INGUINAL NODES

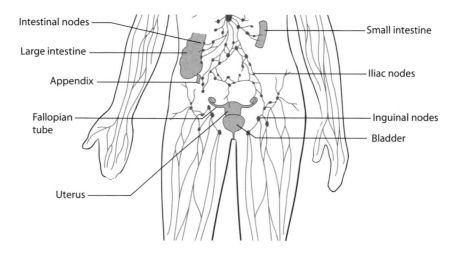

Intestinal nodes

Large intestine

Appendix

Fallopian tube

Uterus

Small intestine

Iliac nodes

Inguinal nodes

Bladder

▲ SIMPLIFIED ILLUSTRATION TO SHOW THE LOCATION OF THE INGUINAL NODES

There are two large collections of lymph nodes in the groin area, known as the inguinal nodes, which are responsible for draining the whole of the leg and part of the lower abdomen. They can easily become overworked dealing with one small infection after another – from bruises or cuts, especially to the leg and insect bites to minor infections such as athlete's foot and leg ulcers – all of which may persist and cause the nodes to become swollen. After a while, the debris generated by chronic, low-grade infection can start to clog up these lymph nodes, causing a variety of apparently unrelated ailments.

One of the general effects of a weakened lymph system is poor healing. Although it can occur in any area where the lymph nodes become congested, this complication is well illustrated by the story of Frederick, whose very problematic recovery was due to a severe obstruction of the inguinal lymph nodes.

Frederick was 19 when he had a nasty accident on his motorbike. The bike was hit by a car and skidded out of control, throwing him off it and landing on top of him. His leg was caught underneath it and he suffered a very bad fracture. Unfortunately he was not wearing proper protective clothing and his skin and tissues were torn away down to the bone as he slid along the surface of the road.

He was in hospital for 18 months, during which time the fracture made very little progress towards healing. The continuing infection prevented the tissues from knitting together and growing over the bone. Consequently, Frederick was facing the possibility of having his leg taken off at the knee.

Frederick's attitude was that he would rather anything than lose his leg, so he decided to discharge himself from hospital and struggle on as best he could. His father phoned me up to ask if there was anything that could be done to assist the healing process. I suggested that they bring him along for a consultation.

The first thing that struck me was that the tissues all looked very unhealthy: the membranes were waterlogged and the wound was discharging some pus and a great deal of blood-stained serum. He also had hugely swollen lymph nodes in his groin. I said that, although I did not hold out a great deal of hope, if I could give him treatment to improve the drainage from the lymph nodes responsible for the damaged area as well as some ultrasonic treatment to the wound itself, then I might bring about some improvement.

After about five weeks of treatment with physiotherapy, the administration of intravenous vitamin B injections plus 1 gram of vitamin C by mouth every day, there was a marked change in the whole picture: the tissues were beginning to look considerably more healthy and healing was underway. After another two or three weeks, the discharge had stopped and the tissues were closing in on the wound. Within a few months of this, skin had begun to grow over the wound. The scar was very ugly-looking, but this was better than having the leg taken off. This all took place six years ago; Frederick has had little further trouble with his leg since then.

ABDOMINAL NODES

The abdominal lymph nodes are rarely given much consideration. You will not usually find them on a diagram of the lymphatic system. Generally speaking, the abdominal lymph nodes do not get obstructed and cause very few problems. The exceptions are the nodes in the lower part of the abdomen, which drain the bladder and uterus. These can become partially blocked – due, most often, to infections of the bladder.

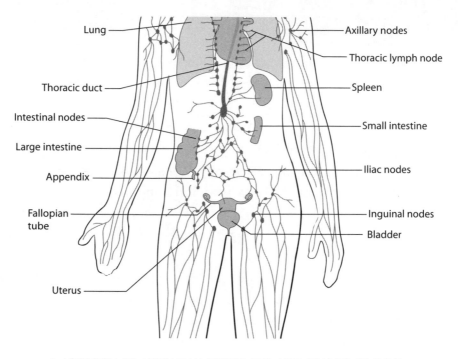

Lung
Axillary nodes
Thoracic lymph node
Thoracic duct
Spleen
Intestinal nodes
Small intestine
Large intestine
Appendix
Iliac nodes
Fallopian tube
Inguinal nodes
Bladder
Uterus

▲ LOCATION OF ABDOMINAL NODES AND AREA DRAINED BY THEM

Infections often get into the bloodstream from our teeth, as the connection between them and the gums is not totally bacteria-proof. Each time you take a bite of food it can cause a shower of bacteria to enter the bloodstream. Normally the bacteria are readily dealt with by filters in the bloodstream, notably the kidneys. They then pass in the urine to the bladder, and from there to the outside world without causing any problems.

Every so often a slightly more powerful bacterium can infect the bladder wall, causing a stream of debris to be dumped in the lymph nodes at the bottom end of the abdominal cavity. These nodes silt up and the lining of the bladder wall then swells, creating conditions which allow much less powerful bacteria to invade – and so the problem is perpetuated.

- Bowel infections do not cause as many problems as bladder infections but can still play a part in congesting the lymph nodes.

- Excessive use of laxatives can also be a contributing factor. They cause a retention of fluid in the large bowel, making conditions more favourable for bacterial growth.

- External infections, particularly of the vulva in women, are a common reason for this blockage.

- There is some intercommunication between the abdominal lymph nodes and those that drain the legs (the inguinal nodes), so an apparently distant infection, such as athlete's foot or cuts shaving may compound the problem.

The abdominal lymph vessels play an important role in the absorption of fats. Fats are large globules which need to be kept from entering the smallest blood vessels, so they are taken into the lymph system and fed into a large lymph duct in the abdomen called the *cysterna chyli*. The intestinal nodes (or Peyer's patches, as they are called) also carry out an important function dealing with most infections of the bowel.

THORACIC NODES

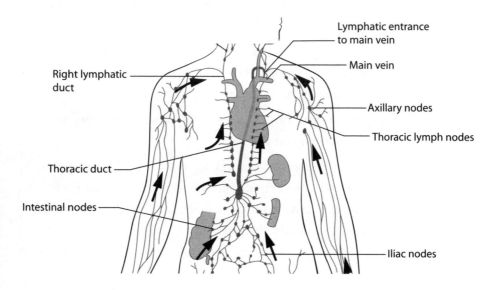

Right lymphatic duct

Thoracic duct

Intestinal nodes

Lymphatic entrance to main vein

Main vein

Axillary nodes

Thoracic lymph nodes

Iliac nodes

▲ SIMPLE DIAGRAM SHOWING LOCATION OF THORACIC NODES AND DRAINAGE ROUTES PLUS KEY ANATOMICAL PARTS

In order to understand how a partial blockage of the thoracic lymph nodes can lead to asthma, bronchitis and other breathing problems, it is helpful to have a basic understanding of how the respiratory system works.

OUR RESPIRATORY TREE

The thoracic lymph nodes are a large group of nodes situated around the point where the windpipe (trachea) divides into the two bronchi which supply the right and left lungs. The bronchi run parallel to the lymph drains and to the blood vessels coming in and out of the lungs, so you have, in effect, four 'trees' going into or coming out of your lungs.

The bronchi branch into smaller and smaller bronchioles which end in the minute air sacs known as alveoli. The air in the alveoli contains oxygen which flows through the alveoli membranes into the blood and is taken up by the red cells. Blood, when it travels back from the tissues to the lungs, contains a high level of carbon dioxide generated by the process of metabolism. This carbon dioxide flows in the reverse direction through the membranes, eventually to be exhaled by the lungs into the atmosphere. The exchange of gases between the air and the blood takes place only in the alveoli, the oxygen actually pushing the carbon dioxide out of the blood.

The surface area of the lungs is so large that, if you were to spread all the alveoli from both lungs out flat, they would occupy the area of a full-size tennis court with all its surrounds.

EXPANDING ALVEOLI

The walls of the alveoli are folded in on themselves, rather like a three-dimensional three-leafed clover, to give the maximum possible surface area for the exchange of gases to take place. In the wall of each alveolus is an elaborate network of arteries, veins and lymphatic vessels, all of which have a different transport function.

The lymphatic vessels carry the lymphatic fluid containing bacteria or viruses and any fluid which may accidentally have passed into the breathing tubes, plus any small particles which may have been inhaled. This fluid travels from the tissue spaces in the wall of the alveoli into the numerous lymph ducts and is carried back to the thoracic lymph nodes at the root of the lung.

The thoracic lymph nodes filter out the solid particles, producing antibodies to combat any infection present and liquefying them or having minute bits engulfed and removed by the white scavenger cells.

A substantial system is needed to service the lungs because the huge surface area exposed to the outside world via the air we breathe can subject it to a risk of massive infection.

OBSTRUCTION OF LYMPH DRAINAGE

As we have seen, the thoracic lymph nodes are positioned around and near the bronchi, so that the smallest blockage is likely to have a major impact on the respiratory system. These nodes may become obstructed for several reasons.

Throughout childhood the lymph nodes are, relatively speaking, in proportion to the rest of the body, so in a very small person they are very small. However, the particles in the air and invading bacteria, always being the same size and thus being relatively much larger in a baby, will clog up the lymph nodes of a child quite easily and, unless treated, this obstruction will continue into adulthood.

8 LIFESTYLE AND LYMPHATIC OVERLOAD

Asthma and Its Treatment

The lymphatic system was designed for the circumstances in which humans evolved. These included unpolluted air, little or no clothing and exposure to only a few varieties of bacteria. Over time, our lifestyles have changed in such a way that the lymphatic system is almost bound to become overloaded.

There has been a huge increase in pollution and in the number of irritating particles in the air. In London very little of the pollution comes from cars. By far the majority is from buses, taxis and lorries which have diesel engines. About three per cent is still industrial pollution. Also there are now many more flowering trees and shrubs in streets and domestic gardens, all of which have pollens which can be irritating; certain crops, like oil seed rape, have aggravating pollen; we now have air conditioning, central heating, fan heaters, double glazing and insulation – so the actual amount and quality of fresh air in the home has dramatically decreased.

As soon as there is a slight chill in the air we tend to close windows and wrap children up in warm clothes. We also travel greater distances and meet many more people, carrying a huge range of infections. This contact with infection is hundreds of times greater than during humanity's early days.

Another facet of modern living that undermines our health in general, and the thoracic lymph nodes in particular, is cigarette smoking.

If you look at the lungs of a smoker, not only are the lungs themselves black with soot, but the thoracic lymph nodes look like little lumps of coal. Smoking seriously contributes to congestion in the lymph nodes, undermining local drainage and weakening resistance to infection. A smoker also exhales millions of particles into the air which are capable of blocking someone else's lymphatic channels.

These modern conditions, sometimes accentuated by food sensitivities, can lead to congestion in the nose and throat area, causing catarrh – often with bacteria present – to drain down the windpipe into the bronchi. From there it may penetrate deep into the lungs, where it is absorbed by the alveoli and some of the small bronchioles and then transported via the lymphatic vessels to the lymph nodes.

This onslaught of catarrh is often too much for the lymph nodes to cope with, and so the debris starts to accumulate, obstructing the passage of fluid through the channels of the lymph nodes and preventing their special cells, the lymphocytes, from making proper contact with any bacteria that have been brought in for disposal. This means that the lymphocytes are not able to form adequate antibodies. As the ability to throw out the current infection is impaired and the resistance to future infections lowered, so the problem is both aggravated and perpetuated.

ASTHMA

Over recent years the number of people suffering from asthma and the severity of the condition have increased alarmingly. In my early days as a doctor, bronchitic asthma was not the life-threatening disease it is today, when it causes between 2,000 and 3,000 deaths a year. In the light of such worrying statistics, it is good to be able to reassure people that most asthma sufferers can be helped to enjoy an active life free from all drugs and sprays.

One child who particularly stays in my mind was five-year-old Bob, a patient at one of my hospitals who was so ill with asthma that he was going to be sent to a special school for invalids.

At the time, Bob was a very sickly boy who suffered badly with bronchitis and asthma. He had been in and out of hospital over the previous two years and his condition was clearly getting worse. The doctors at the hospital were worried and asked if I might be able to help.

When I examined Bob, I found that he had huge lymph nodes in his neck and tremendous spasm and swelling of the tissues in the middle of his thoracic spine, just where the root of the lung comes down. X-rays showed that the lymph nodes located at the point where the windpipe divides into the two bronchi were very waterlogged. I gave Bob treatment to the enlarged lymph nodes in his neck and chest area, and arranged for him to have his unhealthy tonsils removed. After a couple of months Bob's breathing problems started to improve dramatically and the attacks gradually became rare and very mild.

He had an attack of asthma the following year when he caught a cold, and then again two years later after a bout of flu. I gave him more treatment and heard nothing for a few years. Then, one Christmas, his mother sent me a card asking if I remembered her asthmatic son. Well, not only had he been made head boy at school, but he was also captain of the school football and cricket teams and was doing well academically.

Asthma is a curious disease which can be divided into two categories:

1 Allergic asthma – the true disease, which affects about one per cent of asthma sufferers
2 Infective bronchitic asthma – a defence mechanism in response to an infection of the respiratory tract. This response is so exaggerated that it becomes a disease.

These two conditions are both categorized as asthma and often confused with one another. However, it is essential to identify the type of asthma a person is suffering at an early stage so that the correct measures can be taken.

THE ONSET OF ASTHMA

The foundations for bronchitic asthma are very often laid at a young age. Although the hereditary factor does play some part in a child's vulnerability to asthma, the major cause is usually living in an environment which weakens the lymphatic system.

Bronchitic asthma develops in stages and usually has its origins in early childhood. The progression may be something like this: a small baby catches a cold and snuffles a little. Weeks later he catches his next cold and the snuffles intensify. If the nose and mouth are congested, then the catarrhal fluid may go down the bronchial tubes and collect, causing a little rattle in the chest. A further infection causes another rattle in the chest, this time with a wheeze. The next infection brings about the rattle followed by a full-blown spasm of the affected bronchi – the hallmark of the asthmatic condition.

THE PROTECTIVE SPASM

Small children up to the age of about two do not have sufficient co-ordination between their larynx and diaphragm to cough up mucus and other unwanted substances from the bronchial tubes. As they cannot clear them, they do the next best thing – stop these substances getting into the tubes in the first place. This is achieved through a mild protective spasm which may make the child start to wheeze. Air can only get in by the force of atmospheric pressure but is pushed out by the much greater force of the breathing muscles. The tubes are therefore actively dilated to breathe in but tend to collapse on breathing out, hence the wheeze.

If a child's lymphatic system is having to deal with a lot of infection, each time he catches a cold he will start to wheeze. This wheeze will increase with each cold, until the child's conditioned reflexes are so well established that the tubes go into a spasm at the first sign of an infection. This is the start of bronchitic asthma.

The protective mechanism becomes progressively more sensitive until any irritation of the nose (from dust, pollens, animal scurf, moulds, etc.) causes the tubes to go into spasm. Soon only the tiniest particle is needed to trigger the reaction. The situation can reach a point where even going out into cold air can start a spasm. Mild allergies also increase the secretions from the membranes of the nose, throat and sinuses, giving the lung even more fluid to cope with and further aggravating the condition.

If, as a very small child, your tubes go into a spasm when anything irritates your nose or throat, the mechanism becomes so well established that it persists even when you reach the age when you are able to cough up fluid. The tendency for a child to develop asthma as a complication of a chest infection is greatly increased when there is a hereditary factor present. If a relative has asthma, there may also be a copycat effect, as the child learns that this is the normal mechanism for dealing with fluid in the bronchi.

DORMANT PROBLEMS

In some cases, such as Joe's described below, the symptoms of bronchitic asthma may subside for a period of time, then recur later in life.

Joe, who came to see me when he was 27, caught his first bad cold when he was nine months old and had snuffled a great deal. He had had several colds over the next few months, and each time the snuffles got worse. His mother also started to notice a rattle in his chest. When he was two and a half, he had a cold which, predictably, went to his chest. This time, however, he had a spasm of his bronchial tubes – his first attack of bronchitic asthma.

Over the next year or so, Joe went down with more 'chesty' colds, all of which developed into asthma, until the onset of each asthma attack virtually coincided with the start of the cold. By the age of five, exposure to cold air or dust alone was enough to trigger an attack. The colds, however, were beginning to be less frequent and each asthma attack became less severe.

By the time Joe was seven, he had stopped having other than normal colds and the asthma had receded. By the age of 10 it had completely disappeared. This was because his lymphatic system had given him immunities to all the ambient infections. He remained reasonably fit (although not very robust) until he was 24, when he had a bad dose of flu, followed by bronchitis and then a bad attack of asthma. From then on he had attacks of increasing severity – and at decreasing intervals – until he came to me for a consultation.

Sensitivity tests showed a large number of substances to which Joe was mildly allergic. He said that attacks were triggered by cold air, cigarette smoke and other irritating substances, such as dust in the wind. He was very 'chesty'.

On examination, his nose and throat had swollen membranes and there was some discharge from the sinuses running down the back of his throat. I could hear wheezing over a great deal of his lungs, particularly in the lower lobes. There was a number of very large lymph nodes in his neck, especially in the area above his collarbone, and some spasm of the muscles in the chest area of his spine. I noticed considerable waterlogging of the tissues of the back level with the root of the lungs. An x-ray showed a number of enlarged lymph nodes around the root of the lung as well.

Joe received treatment to the lymph nodes in his neck and those near the root of his lung, as well as advice on general health, diet, the importance of fresh air and the consequences of overclothing. After about 15 treatments he was completely free of the asthma and bronchitis. However, as can happen, about four months later he caught a bad cold which brought on an attack, followed by another some eight months later. The last attack was very mild and went off very rapidly.

At his check-up a year later, Joe said he had had no further asthma attacks and was delighted by the fact that he had been the only member of his family not to catch a cold a few weeks before. He also felt much fitter in general following the treatment.

The recurrence of Joe's asthma in his twenties was due to his weakened lymph system. By the age of seven a child's lymphatic system has manufactured antibodies against most of the everyday bacteria that he is likely to come into contact with. With so many circulating antibodies, the young Joe was no longer susceptible to infections and it was generally assumed that he had grown out of the asthma.

However, the blockage in the lymphatic system had not been cleared. While he was very young, fit and resilient, he remained free of trouble. But as he reached his early twenties and his defence mechanism started to weaken a little, the sudden attack of flu overloaded his lymph system and activated the protective spasm, causing a return of the bronchitic asthma.

THE PSYCHOLOGY OF ASTHMA

Although asthma is a physical disease, it also has a psychological side which needs to be borne in mind. For example, a child's subconscious will notice that she was unable to do something she disliked because of an asthmatic attack. With the next unpleasant situation the subconscious will mimic an asthmatic attack as an evasive tactic. Although psychologically triggered, it will be identical to the physical one. The child does not know that it is the subconscious brain that is at work.

This side of asthma needs to be addressed from the outset, as it can become more and more crippling; the slightest thing that the child wants to avoid can bring on an attack. Unfortunately, the brain does not distinguish between something unpleasant and something exciting. When you are looking forward to something, such as a party or a holiday, this stimulates your adrenaline mechanism and makes your pulse race in the same way as it would if you were feeling fear or panic. So the sufferer is just as likely to have an attack when she desperately wants to do something as when she desperately does not.

In extreme cases, children can suffer as many as 10 or more of these psychological attacks for every purely physical one. Clearly, parents need to be firm and ensure that their child leads as normal a life as possible in order to minimize these. It is amazing how quickly the subconscious will stop turning on the attacks if the desired response is denied. This is well illustrated by the story of nine-year-old Joanna.

Joanna was brought to see me because she was having very frequent asthma attacks. I gave her the usual treatment and, although the clinical signs got better (the congestion improved, the lymph nodes decreased in size and her breathing sounded better), the attacks of asthma continued unabated. This was puzzling because there was no obvious explanation.

The first clue came when I asked Joanna what she was going to do after her visit. Her mother said that they would have to hurry back home as her aunt was coming to stay. Joanna threw a great tantrum and insisted that her mother had promised they would go out to lunch. A big argument followed between mother and daughter, suddenly the wheezing started and Joanna was in the middle of a full-blown asthma attack. Her parents looked at each other and concluded that they would have to postpone the aunt coming to stay because they must take their daughter out to lunch. Although they had not promised this treat at all, they felt it might help the asthma.

Next time she came to see me, I said that I wanted to talk to her parents by themselves. This is something that I rarely do, as I think it is important that children know everything that is going on. However, in these particular circumstances it was appropriate. I explained that, although the attacks were genuine, there was obviously a psychological overlay to the condition and that, while Joanna knew they would give in to her every demand under the threat of an asthma attack, they were perpetuating her ill-health.

I stressed that, although it would be traumatic for them, it was important to take a tough line. It was, as the saying goes, a case of being cruel to be kind. Her parents phoned up on several occasions saying that Joanna was not well enough to go to school – what should they do? I repeated that they must harden their hearts and tell the school that the asthma was psychological and it was important that Joanna was not allowed to use it as a way of avoiding things she did not want to do.

They were very distressed, but I reassured them and sympathized, saying that it was probably one of the hardest things that parents could be called upon to do. Once Joanna's parents showed her that they would not respond to the pressure of her psychological attacks, she got much better. She still had the occasional attack, but they gradually faded out and, in the end, she was completely free of the trouble.

TREATMENT OF BRONCHITIC ASTHMA

It is my belief that an asthmatic condition can actually be made worse by modern medicine. The treatment for asthma has changed quite dramatically over the past 50 years or so. At one time only fairly simple drugs such as aminophylline were available for treating a bad attack of asthmatic spasm. In extreme cases an injection of adrenalin would be given, but such treatments could only be administered by a specialized doctor. The aerosols and tablets that are now taken at home on a routine basis were not available.

Nowadays, when a child goes to the doctor with a wheeze, he will sooner or later be prescribed a steroid and/or bronchodilator spray to be used in the event of an attack. As the disease develops, the parents may well be advised to administer these sprays routinely to reduce the child's sensitivity to particles in the air. If the condition becomes altogether worse, pills of a similar nature may also be prescribed as routine medication.

The widespread practice of prescribing cortisone and bronchodilator drugs for asthma sufferers on a relatively long-term basis has many detrimental effects.

■ These drugs reduce the blood supply to the tissues of the bronchi during their active phase by constricting the blood vessels, only to be followed a few hours later by a huge surge of blood to the tissues to compensate for the period of 'starvation'. This brings about the very condition in the body – congestion – which the drugs are trying to relieve, and ensures that they will be needed again to control their own after-effects.

- Steroids lower the child's resistance to infection, as does the increased congestion from the fluctuating blood supply. With every subsequent infection the body grows more sensitive to the reflexes that close down the tubes, and so the asthma becomes more apparent.

- Treatment with cortisone preparations suppresses the body's natural output of cortisol from the adrenal glands, making asthma a potentially life-threatening disease. When I first started practising, doctors firmly believed that, however bad the attack of asthma, at the moment of extreme distress the body would produce a massive output of cortisol and adrenalin to release the spasm. Given their capacity to suppress the body's natural protective reactions, cortisone drugs may well be a factor in the fatal asthma attacks that occur nowadays.

MANAGEMENT OF ASTHMA

The treatment of asthma can be divided into two distinct parts: care during an attack, and management between attacks. If the sufferer has been asthmatic for some time and has been taking steroids or other drugs, then the existing regime should be continued until there is sufficient improvement in the general condition to begin modifying it. If the attack is severe, then it may be necessary to go to hospital. However, I believe that the management of the condition between attacks may require a completely different approach if the patient is to be helped to resume a healthy life without use of drugs.

My recipe for the management of asthma has five different aspects: a change in lifestyle, dietary changes and supplements, reviewing the state of the tonsils, breathing exercises and physical medicine.

Change in Lifestyle

It is very important that asthmatic children and adults should be as fit and hardy as possible. If the lymphatic system is to be restored to full working order, then the huge blood supply in the bronchial tree and in the nose and throat must be allowed to settle down. This means taking the measures described in chapter 4, which include getting plenty of fresh air and exercise and, for children, cutting back on extra layers of clothing, cutting out the heating in bedrooms, and not allowing the condition to stop them leading a normal life.

This advice is not always easy for parents to take – but if they ignore it the patient cannot be expected to get better, as Ian's case demonstrates.

Ian had suffered from asthma since he was three years old. He started out as a healthy baby, but by the age of nine months he was beginning to go down with one cold after another and becoming very snuffly in general. By the time he was 18 months old, each cold he caught was accompanied by bronchitis.

After a few attacks, the bronchitis became wheezy and rapidly turned into asthma. For a year or two the asthma had been brought on by chesty colds. Subsequently it began to be triggered by Ian going out into cold air or into a dusty atmosphere. He was soon having asthma for no apparent reason. When I examined him I found that he had a large number of tender lymph nodes in his neck, extending right down to his collarbone. He had tremendous spasm and swelling in the muscles of his thoracic spine.

Ian's mother said that she could not understand how he could be constantly ill when she looked after him so well. He was never allowed to get cold and was always well clothed. He never went out without some sort of an overcoat. I explained about the consequences of overclothing and how important it was that she and her partner reduce the level of their son's clothing to an absolute minimum. They appeared to understand this and, each time Ian came to me for treatment, he was lightly dressed.

Sadly, however, even with all the treatment and apparent cooperation, Ian's condition didn't improve as much as I had expected. There was clearly something going wrong somewhere. We looked at the treatment again and spent a long time considering this puzzle. However, two visits later, my secretary asked me to look out of the window quickly. Ian had just left through the front door and was being bundled into more and more clothing. He was then driven off in an air conditioned car. It became quite clear why he had not shown the expected improvement.

I had a few words with the parents next time I saw them and the message did eventually get through – and, I am happy to say, Ian started to make great strides. After another couple of months he was much better. However, like many asthma sufferers he was not completely free of attacks for about three years, after which time his resistance to infection had also become formidable.

If parents are able to make the leap of faith and follow these changes through, it is astonishing how a case of bronchitic asthma will resolve itself, as this gratifying story shows:

Two or three years ago my wife and I were emerging from a wedding reception and I hailed a taxi. As we climbed into the taxi the driver asked me if I was a doctor (he recollected that he had picked me up some years previously and taken me to my practice in Devonshire Place). On that occasion, he had told me about his daughter, who had very bad asthma and was spending two or three months every year in hospital on oxygen. As far as he could tell it was steadily getting worse and he and his wife were worried about her future: 'You told me there was a lot one can do oneself about asthma, and gave me advice about clothing, feeding, etc. For the last four

years I have been desperately hoping to pick you up again so that I would
be able to say thank you, as for four years she hasn't had a touch of asthma after taking your advice.'

Dietary Changes – Extra Vitamins

Cow's milk may need to be eliminated for a while and the following
supplements taken. Vitamins A, D and C bolster the body's ability to
resist and throw off infections. Vitamin B helps to boost general well-
being (see page 55).

Check the Tonsils

If the tonsils are infected, they need to be removed. The asthma will
never be overcome if a constant supply of infections and toxins is
being harboured by the tonsils.

**It is important to remember that the appearance of the
tonsils is not as important as the general health of the child
and the state of the tonsil lymph nodes.**

Breathing Exercises

These are very important for asthmatics who, due to the build-up of
catarrhal secretions, tend gradually to reduce the amount of lung that
they use. The lung, like all parts of the body, has a huge and under-
used capacity. It is quite possible living a fairly quiet life to use only a
fifth of the capacity of the lung, but this fifth should change from one
part to another to maintain the health of the lung. A conscious effort
is required to make proper use of the whole lung. Breathing exercises
help to ensure that it is kept in fit condition.

To loosen up the chest and shoulder muscles, inhale with your arms
outstretched and, as you exhale, slowly pull arms backwards and circle
in a clockwise direction five times (see diagram on page 115). Repeat

anti-clockwise. To stretch the upper back and chest, inhale and grasp your hands behind your back, then, as you exhale, lift your arms up and hold until you feel a good stretch in your chest and front shoulder (see diagram below). Repeat five times. Do these stretching exercises at least once a day.

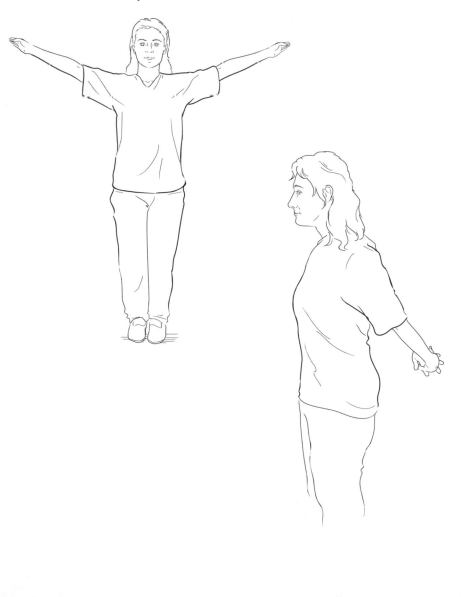

Lie down on a firm surface with a pillow under your head and your knees slightly bent or supported. Place your hands on your abdomen, just below the lower ribs (see diagram below). Breathe in slowly to a count of three and feel your abdomen rise. Breathe out to a count of four and feel it return to normal. Squeeze your abdominal muscles at the end of each outbreath. Repeat five times.

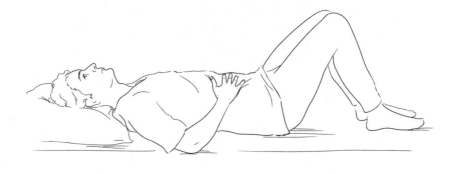

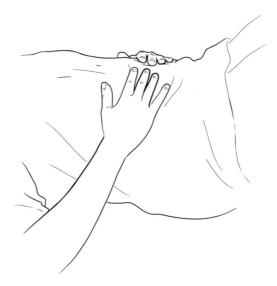

Carry out the same exercise, first with your hands on the sides of your ribs and your fingers pointing inwards, and then with your fingertips resting on your upper chest just below the collarbone (see diagram below). Contract the muscles under your hands to expel the air fully from each part of the lungs. Repeat at least once a day.

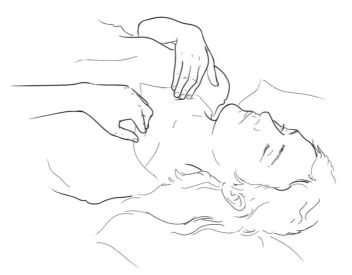

Physical Medicine

This includes massage to the cervical lymph nodes, especially those situated just above the collarbone, and to the thoracic spine (which corresponds to the bra line in women). This area is nearly always rather tight in asthma sufferers. Parents can make an important contribution by doing this.

Ultrasonic waves and electrical treatment applied to the enlarged lymph nodes is also highly beneficial. If the ribs are starting to become stiff, which is fairly common, it is possible to 'mobilize' them using a very simple technique, which improves the breathing capacity of the patient (see Part IV, beginning on page 207, for more details).

On this regime there is usually an improvement within a few weeks. It is then possible to start cutting back on steroids until, eventually, they can be phased out completely. Most children up to the age of 15 will respond readily and show no further signs of asthma. If treated after that age, patients do somewhat less well and, although they should not have serious attacks, they may still have some wheeziness at times. This is especially likely with an infection causing bronchitis.

A–Z DIRECTORY: PROBLEMS ASSOCIATED BY LYMPHATIC MALFUNCTION

ABSCESS, DENTAL

see Dental Problems

ALLERGIES

see Asthma, Food Sensitivities and Hay Fever

APPENDICITIS

The appendix is a small tube two or three inches long which is lined with lymphoid tissue. This lymphoid tissue is responsible for producing antibodies against bacteria. The appendix works flat out in the early years of life to provide immunity against 'bugs' found in the gut so that, in the event of the gut being pierced, there would be a better chance of survival. By the time we are six, the appendix has usually done its job, and ceases to be of any further use.

It can, however, be overwhelmed by bacteria – especially in the presence of tonsillitis, which sets up a drip feed of bacteria via the stomach. When the appendix becomes mildly infected, symptoms include indigestion, alternating diarrhoea and constipation and possibly vague pains. The sufferer may feel under the weather and unusually tired over a period of up to a year or two. Should the infection flare up, it will cause sickness and pain above the navel. These attacks usually subside, but often leave scarring on the appendix.

Eventually, a case of chronic appendicitis (sometimes described as a 'grumbling appendix') will become acute, the bacteria spreading from the wall of the appendix to the peritoneum which covers it. At this point, the pain transfers to the lower right part of the abdomen – **this is a warning sign that you should seek urgent medical attention, as it is life-threatening.** If the pain suddenly vanishes or spreads over the abdomen, the appendix has ruptured. Sudden lack of pain must not be taken as a sign that the condition has gone away – medical help must be obtained.

See also chapter 5.

APPETITE

Left to their own devices, children have an unerring sense of what their body requires. If a child is short of cysteine, for instance, he will often develop an insatiable appetite for eggs, but as soon as the deficiency is made up he will go off eggs and start to seek out foods that address other imbalances. For this reason it is worth paying attention to a child's likes and dislikes. The exception to the rule is sugar, which is not normally available naturally in our diet and, therefore, which most of us seem to find much harder to consume with discrimination and in moderation. Sugar is not a good food and children should be trained to eat as little as possible. Eating food you dislike is of limited benefit, as it does not stimulate the digestive juices effectively. A poor appetite in a child is often due to parents' inflated expectations about what he should be eating. If the unwanted food is taken away from the child and no substitute offered, the child's appetite will usually return.

Overfeeding is surprisingly common. Babies should not necessarily be fat and rounded; leaner children tend to be much more lively and healthy, which is a good thing.

See also chapter 4.

ARTHRITIS

see Rheumatoid Arthritis

ARTHRITIS OF THE OSSICLES

see Ear Problems

ASTHMA

Allergic Asthma

This comparatively rare condition does not fall within the scope of this book. A small minority experience a serious allergic reaction when they breathe in certain substances, which may cause the bronchial tubes to close down. This can be treated by avoidance and desensitization. There's also a new injection which has been tried and is proving successful in treating this condition.

When tests for allergies are carried out on people with bronchitic asthma, the majority turn out to have a number of mild sensitivities, whereas those performed on people with true allergic asthma produce only one or two massive reactions to specific allergens such as cats, dogs, horses or pollens. If you suffer from true allergic asthma then you may be breathing perfectly normally one minute, but as soon as a cat comes into the room you are suddenly fighting for each breath.

This is because your body recognizes the allergen that is inhaled and, however small the actual amount, fears a massive influx. As a result, the whole of the bronchial tree goes into a protective spasm to try to keep the offending substance out. The onset is usually quite sudden; the disease does not come on step by step as the more common, infective version does.

> Allergic asthma and hay fever are close cousins. As the membranes of the bronchial tree are more easily upset than those of the nose, a child tends to react to allergens first with asthma and then, a few years later in life, with hay fever. Some, of course, may only have hay fever.

Infective Bronchitic Asthma or Bronchitis

Bronchitis means inflammation of the bronchus, or breathing tube. Although the symptoms of bronchitic asthma may appear to be similar to those of allergic asthma, the two illnesses have very different causes. Bronchitic asthma arises in response to one of the following:

- a continuous infection caused by a low-grade bacterium which just manages to infect the breathing tube, triggering the secretion of mucus when it goes into an acute phase, to wash the organism away

- a momentary, virulent infection which invades the breathing tubes, causing them to become inflamed and produce a large quantity of mucus.

Bronchitic asthma is a condition which is acquired as a response to mucus in the breathing tube. It may involve only the lower parts of the lung at first, as the mucus tends to drain into them. As it progresses, however, more and more of the lung is affected until eventually the whole bronchial tree may go into spasm during an attack. This type of asthma brings into play a defence mechanism which is particularly active in small children.

When there is an infection in your nose and throat, the membranes that line the upper respiratory tract become inflamed and increase the amount of mucus they secrete. Because these secretions run down into your windpipe there is always a risk that the mucus and debris caused by the infection may enter your lungs. In order in prevent this, the breathing tubes constrict and go into a protective spasm. This is particularly important in the very young, when the ability to cough things out has not been developed.

This reaction usually becomes so exaggerated that the effect of the spasm is more of a problem than whatever it is defending against. Unfortunately, by the time the child has learned to cough, the reflex or habit of the bronchial spasm has become firmly established and so persists into adolescent and adult life.

This type of asthma is very much more common than allergic asthma and can be alleviated by measures taken at home – including, in more severe cases, treatment to restore proper lymphatic drainage through the cervical and thoracic lymph nodes (see page 100). However, if the treatment is to be successful the parents and, where possible, the patient must play a large part in the regime of recovery (see chapter 7 for more information).

Pollen and pollution are often named as causes of asthma, whereas I am convinced that, in the majority of cases, they can only aggravate asthma when it is already present. If they were capable of causing asthma, virtually everyone would suffer, especially those living in cities or large towns.

See also Bronchitis, Emphysema, Hay Fever and chapter 8.

ATHLETE'S FOOT

Almost all fungi love dark, damp, warm conditions, which is why fungal infections flourish around the feet. Shoes and socks have the effect of weakening and dampening the skin of the feet, particularly between the toes. The spores of the fungi that cause athlete's foot circulate in the air, but are also found on any floor or carpet a sufferer has trodden on with bare feet, and readily spread to the softened toes of a new host. The infection is often present for months or even years, but if the soggy, heaped up skin becomes sufficiently weakened it can crack, allowing bacteria to infect it as well.

Over a period of time the huge quantities of debris generated by such an infection pass up to the inguinal nodes in the groin, sometimes causing them to become very overloaded. Treating the actual infection can provide long-term relief if all the organisms and their spores are effectively killed off and no new infection is encountered.

Treatment to the lymph nodes with massage and ultrasonic waves will help provide a permanent remedy for athlete's foot. Massage at home can also be helpful in combating the infection. One reason the condition recurs is that the blocked lymph nodes reduce a person's resistance; thus a cycle is set up. By decongesting the lymph nodes and giving a local fungal treatment to the athlete's foot, it is possible to eliminate the infection once and for all.

Maria, 17, loved sports of all kinds. She was, however, concerned about her very smelly feet. This had become something of a joke at school, so she had been to see a doctor about it when she was 12. The doctor had diagnosed athlete's foot. Maria had tried various local creams and powders and followed advice about cleanliness and, although the condition virtually disappeared for periods of time, it had always broken down again. She came to me to see whether I could get a more permanent result.

On examination, Maria had very large lymph nodes in both sides of her groin. It was my belief that these were interfering with the drainage from her foot, keeping the skin slightly swollen and weakening her resistance. This allowed the spores or fungus to retain a foothold (as it were!) and to multiply when the opportunity arose.

Maria had 11 treatments in all to these lymph nodes, after which they were greatly reduced in size. She also had a further course of pills for athlete's foot and some ointment to put between her toes, which cleared the condition permanently.

BEHAVIOURAL PROBLEMS

See Psychological Problems, and chapter 5.

BELL'S FACIAL PALSY

The main symptoms of this condition are a drooping (on one side only) of the corner of the mouth, the lower eyelid and, to a lesser extent, the facial muscles. It can occur quite suddenly, when the facial nerve is compressed, causing the loss of movement in one side of the face.

The facial nerve is large and important, running in a narrow bony canal across the top of the middle ear. It controls the muscles of facial expression and taste. If the membranes lining the middle ear swell, the lining of the nerve canal may also become swollen, preventing impulses from running down to the face.

In many instances the condition, most commonly brought on by a draught or a bad cold, is temporary. As soon as the cold clears up and the associated swelling goes down, the nerve function is restored. However, if the drainage from the lymph nodes is very poor the swelling will remain and the patient will be left with a permanent weakness in the facial muscles on one side.

It can be most distressing, as the story of Jasmine, aged 33, illustrates:

Jasmine was suffering from a very slight cold when she woke up to discover that the left side of her face had gone lop-sided. Her mouth and her top eyelid on the left side were drooping, but the weakness in the lower lid meant that she could not shut her eye and the muscles of her face had gone completely flaccid. Although the sensation in her face was normal, all the muscles that moved her face on the left side had virtually stopped working.

The condition improved a little over the following weeks and she recovered some movement, but her eye and the corner of her mouth, which dribbled, worried her considerably. She was, understandably, very concerned about her appearance.

On examination, the ear drum in her left ear looked very catarrhal and was somewhat retracted. The drum was also rather red as there was an increased blood supply across it. The muscles of her face were almost completely paralysed, although most of them demonstrated a small amount of movement.

Jasmine received 17 treatments, at the end of which the movement in her facial muscles was about 80 per cent restored. I saw her again two months later for a check-up and the facial palsy could hardly be noticed except when she made certain expressions. In a further two months the problem had entirely resolved.

The orthodox treatment for those cases that do not fully recover is to support structures which have sagged using tape or clips to prevent permanent stretching while the muscles are unable to function. Muscle-tightening operations can also be performed.

A more effective result is obtained by treatment to clear the drainage through the lymph nodes. As it is difficult to get to the site of the actual trouble in the canal, electrical treatment is almost always needed. This is particularly important as the time element is so crucial: the longer the nerve is compressed the more likely it is to become permanently damaged.

About nine months to a year after an attack, the nerve can start to die from the pressure exerted on it. Although it is still possible to relieve the pressure, you can never restore a dead nerve associated with the brain. As long as treatment is given in time, the problem can usually be reversed.

BLEPHARITIS

see Eye Conditions

BLOCKED TEAR DUCTS

see Eye Conditions

BODY TEMPERATURE

The efficient human muscles generate a great deal of heat and, when primitive man shed his 'fur', we developed a new mechanism of cooling our bodies, involving evaporation of fluid from the pores of our skin by sweating. If our bodies are overclothed to such an extent that this mechanism is seriously interfered with, ill-health can result.

Many children are overclothed. Babies should feel warm from the back of the neck down, but there is no need to worry about hands and feet. Older children know if they are cold. The emphasis should be on layers of light clothing. Carrying a pullover or overcoat in case the child feels cold is also a good idea.

We also sweat out salts from the circulation and, if this is excessive, the resulting salt depletion can put us at risk of heat exhaustion or, even more seriously, heatstroke. It is a good idea to take a sachet of salts such as Dioralyte every day when in a hot country to maintain healthy electrolyte levels.

See also chapter 4.

BREASTFEEDING

Breastfeeding is of vital importance in the first few days of life, as it provides a baby with antibodies and special milk. Breastfeeding is also of value later on, when so many children experience difficulties tolerating cow's milk. Cot deaths are generally more common in babies who have been transferred to cow's milk, whereas there are relatively few instances of cot deaths among children who are breastfed for the first few months.

BRONCHITIS

Catarrhal Conditions

Catarrhal conditions involve swelling and inflammation of the mucous membranes, causing an increase in the amount of mucus secreted. The nose, middle ear and sinuses are most commonly affected. They are often due to overheating. If a child is wearing too many clothes or if the room temperature is too hot, the body tends to switch the blood supply from the skin to the throat. Since humans are adapted to cooling their body temperature via the skin, the throat is unable to cope with the increased circulation and merely becomes congested, which leads to catarrh. As one infection follows another, the lymph nodes become partially blocked, causing back pressure and greatly aggravating the catarrhal condition. Food sensitivities can also be responsible.

See also Asthma, Emphysema.

CATARACTS

see Eye Conditions

CELLULITE

Cellulite is the laying down of fat in subcutaneous tissues in blobs, so that it forms little ridges and dimples. It is much more common in women because of physiological differences between the sexes. In a man, one of the secondary sexual characteristics is for the muscles to be covered by a sheath pulled in tightly at the sides, to make the muscles stand out from each other. Women's muscles, on the other hand, were made smooth and rounded by a layer of fat in the subcutaneous tissues, especially on their limbs.

Fat is continuously laid down and taken up by the body. In areas where the circulation is good, such as the neck and face, this can happen very quickly, whereas on the thighs and abdomen it is a much slower process. This explains why someone who has been on a radical diet can look thin and drawn about the face, while there is very little change in the shape of her hips and thighs. Gradual weight loss over a period of time ensures that fat from this area is picked up at the same speed as from the upper body.

If the lymphatic drainage from the skin of the thighs is poor, fat is not always laid down evenly and the typical 'orange peel effect', or cellulite, results. Once the circulation to the area is improved, however, the excess fat which causes this effect will be removed, evening out the coverage and smoothing out the thighs.

Firm massage, both in the direction of the inguinal nodes in the groin and of the nodes themselves, can definitely help to shift stubborn deposits of cellulite by breaking up the fat and improving lymphatic drainage from the thighs. Fat globules are transported by the lymphatic system, so the increased blood supply increases the efficiency of this process as well.

This treatment can remove quite serious cellulite in 10 to 20 visits. Results are even more decisive if the patient eats a balanced, low-fat diet. Drinking 2 litres of water a day will also help to wash the globules of fat into the lymphatic system and so speed up the process.

CEREBRAL OEDEMA

Cerebral oedema is mild fluid retention in the brain, sometimes due to impaired lymphatic drainage. Recurrent throat infections can partially obstruct the lymph nodes in the neck, and since the same lymph nodes drain the brain, the slightest obstruction may result in the brain becoming slightly waterlogged.

Symptoms include abnormal tiredness, a poor short-term memory, very limited powers of concentration and, in children, aggression and a poor response to discipline. Treatment to the lymph nodes and removal of the tonsils – if they are badly infected – will often bring about a marked change in disposition.

CONJUNCTIVITIS

see Eye Conditions

CONSTIPATION

This usually occurs when the diet contains insufficient bulk to stimulate the bowel to expel the faeces, or insufficient water to soften it. As the faeces gradually go hard, they become more and more difficult to expel. For immediate relief I recommend a light laxative such as Senocot (made from senna) which stimulates the large bowel only. If the constipation persists, a glycerin suppository will draw moisture into the bowel, helping to soften the motion and make it easier to expel as well as stimulating the bowel with the increased bulk. If all else fails, an enema may be required.

Having managed the immediate crisis, it is important to ensure that plenty of roughage is included in the diet and at least six glasses of pure water consumed every day. Small quantities of Senocot or prunes may be required for a while to keep the bowels moving. Once the habit is re-established, these can be stopped.

A diet which relies heavily on fast food and pre-prepared meals will not have the necessary bulk content to maintain healthy bowel movements. Regular exercise also helps to stimulate the bowel.

COT DEATH

I have been involved with several cot deaths, including that of my own son, and am convinced that both overheating in children and an intolerance to cow's milk often play a part.

A very small baby will sometimes produce a slight rattle in his chest as he breathes. At this early stage, the fluid will most likely drain into the lymphatic vessels and the rattle will soon clear. However, if the child is living in overheated conditions which weaken his lymphatic system (see chapter 4), the snuffles are likely to increase in frequency and intensity, setting up a continuous flow of fluid into the bronchial tubes. The bronchial tubes themselves may also increase their secretions in response to this constant irritation, further exacerbating the situation.

This rattle on the lungs normally occurs from around one or two months until 18 months of age. It does not impede the child's breathing, but you can hear the fluid moving around the lung area. In my opinion, this rattle should be taken very seriously in the first few months of a child's life, because the fluid contains mucus which has the potential to cause a serious blockage of the airways.

What happens is that, as air is breathed in and out, the fluid content of the mucus evaporates and it becomes thicker, creating a real risk that a lump will travel down and plug one of the narrower breathing tubes. In extreme cases, the thick mucus can completely block off a large part of the lung, which may lead to a cot death. The picture of asphyxiation in cot deaths is almost identical to that caused by an infection. At post mortem, the children are often thought to have had an acute pulmonary infection.

This was what happened to my own baby son, Mark. When he died, a plug of solid mucus resembling a cast of the bronchial tree was pulled out of his lungs. I firmly believe that, if parents listened for the rattle and took action to eliminate the mucus, then cot deaths would be a much rarer thing. You can expel the mucus at home, by holding your child upside down and giving the ribs a little squeeze – or ask your doctor or health visitor to do it for you. Once it has been eliminated, it is important to address the cause of the problem – the diet (especially cow's milk), over-clothing and over-heating.

COW'S MILK

Cow's milk is not an essential part of a child's diet (see chapter 4). If it is required, it can be given for the first few months, but babies can usually be weaned fairly early onto ordinary food and drink (water and fruit juices) and often benefit from this, as so many of them have some degree of intolerance to cow's milk. This intolerance can cause a variety of problems including catarrhal conditions, eczema and digestive problems.

CYSTITIS

If the lymph nodes in the lower part of the abdomen are congested, it can cause the membrane lining the bladder to become swollen, leaving it much more vulnerable to bacterial attack and infection. This condition is known as cystitis.

Cystitis begins with an urgent need to pass urine at frequent intervals. As the infection spreads to the urethra, passing urine becomes more and more painful until it reaches the point where many sufferers say that it is like passing gravel or ground glass.

The standard treatment is to take substances that control the acidity of the urine, since the infecting bacteria do not like alkaline (non-acidic) conditions. In more severe cases, antibiotics are often prescribed. However, this does not always get to the root of the problem and so the cystitis keeps recurring.

Mary was 37 and came to me because she was suffering from so many headaches. She had been investigated for various conditions – her eyes had been tested, she had had a neurological examination – and nothing abnormal had been found.

When I looked at her I noticed that she had a rather stiff neck and felt tenderness under her skull bone. This is a very common cause of headaches and offered a satisfactory explanation for why they were occurring. After two treatments Mary said that the headaches were getting better, but then added that the real trouble was her 'waterworks'.

She told me that she lived her life darting from one lavatory to another, and had familiarized herself with the whereabouts of all the public conveniences on every route she went on so she could plan her day. The frequency and urgency of her visits were spoiling her life.

Her doctor agreed to refer her to me for treatment, as all his efforts had failed to provide permanent relief. I examined her abdomen and discovered that the bladder area was extremely sensitive to the touch. Her abdominal lymph nodes were also enlarged and tender. I suggested that she had originally had one acute infection and that this had overloaded her lymph nodes and caused the membrane of her bladder to become slightly swollen.

As a result, every time bugs were filtered out of the blood by the kidneys, they settled in the wall of the bladder and so the trouble continued. As a result of the poor lymphatic drainage, the antibody response to these bacteria was very inadequate, which undermined her ability to resist and overcome the infection.

Mary had ultrasonic treatment to the abdominal lymph nodes and to the bladder itself on 15 occasions at increasing intervals. By the end of the treatment the act of passing urine had become much less painful and she was able to last for periods of up to an hour without having to go to the lavatory. Although it was an improvement, it was still far from being a marvellous result.

The lymph nodes were so much reduced in size that I did not feel further treatment would serve any purpose, so I suggested a three-month gap before reassessing both the cystitis and the headaches. When Mary came back, she reported that there had been a steady improvement and she could now last for two to three hours between visits to the lavatory. She was finally able to face long journeys and visits to the cinema. After six months, her condition remained stable.

The main treatment for cystitis is massage to the lymph nodes in the groin area, particularly on the abdominal side of the inguinal ligament, which runs from the pubis to the pelvic bone (see diagram on page 223). The other lymph nodes in the groin may also need massaging, as they are responsible for draining some of the lower parts of the bladder and urethra.

Massage can be given at home to the lymph nodes in the groin area, but the abdominal nodes are situated too deep in the abdomen to receive any real benefit from massage. Ultrasonic waves are used over the enlarged lymph nodes, together with electrical muscle stimulation to the small of the back, as this tends to improve the circulation. Interferential electricity aimed at the base of the bladder can also have a powerful decongesting effect.

In order to regulate the acidity of the urine, potassium citrate tablets are recommended. These make conditions in the bladder unfavourable for the bacteria, and the urine less irritating to the bladder. Patients are advised to drink a lot of water, unless they are taking antibiotics, in which case the urine needs to be reasonably concentrated to increase the antibiotics' effect. It is also advisable to avoid vaginal deodorants.

DEAFNESS

see Ear Problems

DENTAL PROBLEMS

Brushing the gums rather than teeth with a fairly stiff brush will improve the seal between the gums and the teeth, strengthen the gums themselves, and help to prevent the gums from receding. Good brushing habits also improve the circulation to and lymphatic drainage from the gums, which provides some protection against dental infection.

A surprising number of people suffer from mild scurvy because of a vitamin C deficiency, which is bad news for teeth and gums alike. Make sure your diet includes food which demands vigorous chewing to work the roots of your teeth and even out the grinding surfaces.

Dental abscesses can be helped by massaging the lymph glands under the chin and jawbone, in the direction of the larynx. This should be done for several minutes once or twice a day. Ultrasonic waves to the same lymph nodes and to the tooth itself from outside the cheek will also eliminate an infection more quickly.

DIARRHOEA

see Irritable Bowel Syndrome

DIZZINESS

see Ear Problems

DOLPHINS

Dolphins emit a very high-frequency sound wave which bounces back off objects, giving them information about their surroundings and allowing them to communicate with other dolphins. This sound wave can also be used to stun the creatures they wish to catch, including sharks. We use a similar sort of sound wave, called an ultrasonic wave, in medicine to speed up the repair mechanism and draw the swelling out of inflamed or congested areas. It is now thought likely that dolphins, who can be rather belligerent creatures, are friendly to humans because their sonar allows them to visualize our skeleton, which they then recognize as that of fellow mammals.

This same penetration could easily lie behind the beneficial effect that dolphins seem to have on humans, especially those with special needs. Their built-in sonic device endows them with a natural healing and decongesting capacity which may explain the immense sense of well-being that humans experience after contact with these creatures.

DOWAGER'S HUMP

At around 50 or 60 years of age, the thoracic curve in the back sometimes becomes more accentuated, particularly in women. There is also a pad of tissue at the top of the thoracic spine which stands out, often referred to as Dowager's Hump. It may accompany a level of osteoporosis and calcium deficiency, so both of these should be checked.

Although it is generally thought to be a pad of fat, I have found that when you apply pressure to the tissue with a thumb, it leaves an indentation, which suggests that it is filled with fluid. Dowager's Hump is usually regarded as a very difficult condition to treat, but lymphatic drainage, especially if it is combined with hormone replacement therapy and manipulation to mobilize the thoracic spine and reduce the curvature, can bring about a great improvement and even a total cure of this problem.

It should be noted that any food sensitivities, especially for coffee, can increase the tendency to retain fluid and so great care should be taken with the diet during and after treatment. Some people notice that they need to empty their bladder more frequently than usual for a while after the treatment. This is almost certainly an indication of the amount of fluid being removed from the tissues.

EAR PROBLEMS

Middle Ear Infection

Infections travelling up the Eustachian tube from the throat (see diagram on page 85) can result in catarrhal conditions of the middle ear, a perforated drum, or glue ear. In its mildest form, this may involve a degree of deafness, mainly in relation to high notes, and a feeling of discomfort in the ear. This is often a long-standing condition and is more commonly found in adults.

As in the nose, a more virulent ear infection produces a discharge, which can vary from a watery fluid to thick mucus. Unlike the nose, however, the fluid in the middle ear only has the thin Eustachian tube to drain through and, if the mucus is thick and the membranes lining the Eustachian tube swollen, it may not be able to pass. If it is allowed to accumulate, the pressure within the middle ear will build up and eventually the eardrum will burst, producing a discharge.

If a diagnosis is made early enough, it is definitely preferable for a surgeon to make a slit in the ear to release the pressure, because, if the drum is allowed to burst, it may occur in a place that will not repair so easily.

Middle ear infections used to be very serious and distressing before the introduction of antibiotics. For some people, however, they are still a recurrent problem.

Lucy was nearly eight years of age. When she was four, she'd had a sore throat and some ear trouble and then seemed quite healthy until the following winter, when she had two more sore throats and, again, rather bad earache. The next year her left ear began to secrete a discharge and she felt very unwell. An ear, nose and throat surgeon removed her tonsils and there was some improvement, but she still had a tendency to catch a lot of colds and, each time, suffered a discharge from her ear.

Lucy had intermittent trouble and was given several courses of antibiotics, but the condition did not clear for long. She was eventually brought to me. She had very hard, large lymph nodes in her neck as a result of these old infections. I gave her treatment on 14 occasions over a period of four months, at the end of which her lymph nodes had gone down and her ear condition had greatly improved, although it was still not under control. It took about six months for her ear to settle down completely after the treatment and, since then, her general health and resistance to infection has gone from strength to strength.

> When the middle ear itself becomes infected or is being upset by tonsil or throat infections, antibiotics are required to eliminate the problem as quickly as possible and to prevent this part of the ear from being further damaged by successive attacks.

Most of the problems that plague the middle ear are due, directly or indirectly, to an imbalance of pressure between the air outside and inside the middle ear. As we have seen, this pressure is normally equalized by the Eustachian tube, but if the membranes lining this small tube are swollen, then it can become partially or, less often, completely blocked. Treatment to the lymph nodes in the throat (see page 218) will generally clear the problem. Quite often, damaged tonsils continue to inflame the area, making the membranes swell. If this is so, then the tonsils and adenoids should be removed.

Glue Ear

A discharging ear is one of nature's solutions to the problem of pressure in the middle ear. The alternative is that the mucus accumulates in the middle ear and becomes thicker and thicker, until it starts to resemble glue. This sticky substance interferes with the movement of the eardrum and minute bones of the middle ear, causing deafness. This condition is known as glue ear.

The traditional treatment is for a doctor to insert a grommet – a small plastic tube the size of a split pea – into the outer eardrum to enable the gluey mucus to drain out, air to enter and the bones of the ear to move freely. The grommet is designed to come out of its own accord – usually after about six months – once the immediate condition is resolved. If not, it can be removed from the drum.

A grommet is a very useful device as the 'glue' is too thick for the natural defences of the body to absorb. This needs to be followed by treatment to the lymph nodes to ensure that the Eustachian duct remains unobstructed and any fluid that does collect can escape while it is still liquid enough so to do.

Arthritis of the Ossicles

The three bones of the middle ear (the ossicles) are connected to each other by tiny joints to allow ease of movement with minimal friction.

Because these joints transmit sound, they are almost continuously moving and so are subject to a lot of wear and tear.

Normally joints repair themselves as they go, so that they end the day in the same condition as they started. However, if the repair mechanism is upset by catarrh or poor tissue circulation, then arthritis may set in. The arthritis will start in a very mild form, but then the body tries to bolster up the damaged joints by increasing their size with extra bone. This has a similar effect to welding a lump of metal on the hinge of a door to make it stronger. Unfortunately, the door will no longer open properly as it compresses the lump of metal. Increased bone around a joint similarly diminishes its range of movement.

In terms of hearing, the arthritis manifests itself initially as an inability to respond to the considerable movement required for the transmission of bass notes, resulting in low note loss of hearing. However, the waterlogging of the membranes due to the swelling also interferes with the transmission of the very fast moving high notes.

William, 34, said that he had suffered a lot of colds in his early years and was still a bit catarrhal, but had kept fairly well for the past 15 years. He had had the occasional sore throat and caught a few colds, but that was all. However, he had noticed that he was not hearing very well. He had his ears tested and was told that he had loss of both the low and high note range.

When I examined William, I saw that his eardrums were rather dull. Healthy eardrums are shiny and, if a light is shone in the ear, they reflect it back. The membrane lining his nose was a little swollen and there was some discharge present. There were a number of enlarged lymph nodes in both sides of his neck. I decided that the joints in the bones of the middle ear had gone a bit stiff and that this was interfering with the conduction of sound, especially with the bass notes.

William had treatment to the lymph nodes in his neck and gradually his hearing got better. There was an improvement of about 60 per cent over a period of two months. He came to see me again three months later and had four more treatments to his lymph nodes, which were still somewhat enlarged. His hearing improved marginally at this time, but when I saw him three months after that it had become considerably better.

After three more treatments the lymph nodes were still not completely normal, but we agreed that the amount of treatment that would be required to obtain a perfect result was not really justified. I saw William finally six months later, when his condition had become stable and his hearing almost restored to normal.

Orthodox treatment is usually concerned with clearing up the catarrh, first by removing tonsils and adenoids if these are infected and, secondly, with either pills or sprays to dry up the mucus. Surgical treatment to the joints of the ossicles can often effect a considerable improvement. However, treatment to restore drainage through the lymph nodes, which clears the Eustachian tube and improves the tissue circulation and health of the middle ear, will usually relieve the problem on a more permanent basis. It is often helpful to apply electrical muscle stimulation to the facial nerve, as this greatly improves the drainage away from the ear.

Inner Ear Conditions

The inner ear is made up of three separate devices, all forming cavities serviced by the inner ear fluid. If the drainage from the lymph nodes in the neck – especially those located under the ear – is poor, it presents an obstacle to the drainage of fluid from the inner ear. The fluid may also thicken, giving rise to inflammation and irritation of these very delicate pieces of apparatus.

The lymph nodes in the neck can be decongested at home using the massage techniques described on page 215, but electrical stimulation to the muscles of the face may also be of benefit.

Deafness and Dizziness

If the drainage from the inner ear is impaired, this can lead to a low-grade catarrhal condition in the semi-circular canals. One effect of this is that the membrane secretes a thicker fluid which does not stay put as the head is moved. The brain therefore receives faulty messages from the balance mechanism, which tells it that the head is stationary when it is moving.

In other words, the movements of the head are wrongly interpreted by the brain and this results in the person feeling dizzy. The sensation is as though the room were spinning round, in the same way that when a train on an adjacent platform is moving off in the opposite direction, you think that your train is pulling out of the station, although you are standing still.

Alison, aged 38, had had her first attack of dizziness two years earlier. She caught an abnormally large number of colds and most of these were accompanied by earache, particularly in her left ear. On three occasions there was some discharge from her ear, but this had rapidly cleared with the use of antibiotics. The most distressing symptom had started about six months later, when she suddenly found the room spinning around as she tried to stand up.

Alison had five further similar attacks, the last two within a few weeks of each other. Her ears had been investigated and it was found that the balancing mechanism of her ears – the semi-circular canals – was slightly catarrhal. This was making her body think that she was falling one way, an error which her brain immediately corrected, creating the sensation in Alison's head that the room was spinning around.

On examination, Alison had a number of enlarged hard lymph nodes in her neck. These were treated on 17 occasions, at the end of which they had virtually disappeared and she had stopped having dizzy spells. She had only two more, mild and short-lived attacks – one when she went down with a bad cold about five months later, and the other about two months after that when she caught a mild dose of flu.

It was fortunate for Alison that she came for treatment before the condition had become too advanced. As time goes on, the inflammation of the semi-circular canals can result in the sensitive hairs in the cochlea becoming less effective, leading to varying degrees of hearing loss.

Caroline, aged 39, came to see me because she was plagued by colds and was very catarrhal. In the previous few years she had been experiencing a lot of earache as well. More recently she was very disturbed because she seemed to be becoming rather deaf. On examining her I discovered that Caroline's nose was full of discharge and the membranes were a little swollen. There was also some discharge dripping down the back of her throat.

Caroline's eardrums were very dull, with a whitish tinge, which showed that they were full of fluid. The drums were also pushed inwards by the pressure of the air on the outside, and so tightly stretched across the bone which joins onto the drum that they were moulded around it. She had a large number of hard lymph nodes which could be felt on both sides of her neck, particularly on the left side.

I decided that there were probably three reasons for her deafness:

1 the drum was not transmitting sound effectively
2 the tiny ossicles, or bones, were being compressed by the drum, reducing their ability to transmit sound from the outer to the inner drum
3 there was some catarrh in the membranes of the middle and inner ear.

Caroline had treatment to the lymph nodes in her neck and to the drainage channels leading from her ear, and recovered about two-thirds of her hearing. More significantly, there was no further deterioration in her hearing in the next year or so.

Another consequence of this catarrhal condition is an increased blood supply to the area, which can lead to noises in the ear, or *tinnitus*.

Tinnitus

When poor drainage upsets the circulation in a particular area of the body, it is compensated for by nature making an attempt to improve local conditions with an increase in the blood supply to the affected part. This is to correct the lack of adequate supplies and relieve the build-up of waste products. In the case of the ear, some of the increased blood supply runs through the minute blood vessels across the eardrum, and the speed of the flowing blood can sometimes reach such a pitch that it can actually be heard. This distressing condition is known as tinnitus.

Sufferers complain of rushing, squeaking and other strange noises – sometimes continuously, sometimes at intervals. The apparent sound can vary considerably because the actual flow and the number of vessels open varies, but the single most significant factor is the tension of the drum itself. One of the miracles of many of our senses is that they cover a greater range of sensitivity than might normally seem possible. Take the ear: it can hear a faint whisper, but can also cope with the crash of a full orchestra.

The ear achieves this ability to cover such a variety of sound by a very simple device. If the environment is deathly quiet, then a muscle attached to the edge of the drum contracts, stretching the drum extremely tight. This allows it to respond to the most minute vibration. If you are at a noisy party, then the muscle slackens off and the drum becomes relaxed; it will now only be able to respond to a fairly loud wave. There is, of course, every gradation of control in between. It is for this reason that noises in the ear are particularly troublesome in a quiet environment and less noticeable in a crowd.

The usual treatment for tinnitus is to give a drug called Serc (generic name betahistine). This improves the blood supply to the whole of the ear and, in some cases, by increasing the resistance to infection can reduce the catarrhal condition and the 'ringing' sensation. Tinnitus is a notoriously difficult problem to treat and most people have to resign themselves to living with this distressing condition. However, I have found that treatment to restore normality to the lymph drainage will often allow the blood supply to normalize, largely relieving the tinnitus and transforming the patient's quality of life. The condition can also be helped greatly by training the brain to ignore the tinnitus and concentrate on the wanted sound instead.

Treatment is very similar to that required for the middle ear. However, if the muscles at base of the neck are in spasm they may also need attention, as the resulting congestion can have the effect of upsetting the *stellate ganglion*, a 'computer' that controls the circulation to the ear.

Gordon, aged 63, had heard noises in his ears for about three years. He first noticed a high-pitched whistle, which had only lasted for a short time. At first, he thought it was some external noise and searched around for the source, but when other people assured him that they could not hear anything strange, he realized that it was coming from his own hearing mechanism.

After a few months he heard the whistling sound again, this time followed by rushing noises. A few weeks later he found that the rushing noises started up every morning and went on during the day. Sometimes they cleared, sometimes they remained. Gradually the squeaks and rushing noises became more or less constant. Gordon said that he found that if he was in a crowd with a lot of noise then the sounds were minimal, but if the surroundings were very quiet they then became very loud and obtrusive. They were beginning to interfere with his well-being and were especially bad at night.

On examination, both of his eardrums appeared slightly retracted and red, the left more than the right. He had a number of enlarged lymph nodes in his neck, but nothing much else to show. Gordon did have slight trouble at the base of his neck from an old injury.

Gordon underwent treatment to the lymph nodes, first twice a week, then at weekly intervals, and finally every two weeks. After 16 visits the noises were beginning to subside and he was having several hours a day when he heard no noises at all.

I saw Gordon three months later and, although the noises had not ceased entirely, they were becoming much less distressing. I gave him two more treatments and asked to see him again in three months, by which time the noises had become even less intrusive. However, he phoned shortly afterwards to say that he had had another cold and the problem had intensified. I told him to take antihistamine drugs; the condition settled down fairly well. After another three months, Gordon said that the noises had largely cleared.

The more recent and intermittent the problem, generally the easier it is to clear up. Although it is not possible to help all cases of tinnitus,

around 70 per cent can be greatly improved by lymphatic treatment (see Part IV).

Menière's Disease

If you are unfortunate enough to be affected by dizzy spells, increasing deafness and noises in the ear at the same time, then the condition is known as Menière's disease. The symptoms are often short-lived and intermittent at first, but the noises and the deafness tend gradually to become permanent as the disease progresses.

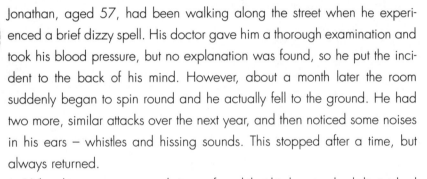

Jonathan, aged 57, had been walking along the street when he experienced a brief dizzy spell. His doctor gave him a thorough examination and took his blood pressure, but no explanation was found, so he put the incident to the back of his mind. However, about a month later the room suddenly began to spin round and he actually fell to the ground. He had two more, similar attacks over the next year, and then noticed some noises in his ears – whistles and hissing sounds. This stopped after a time, but always returned.

When his ears were tested, it was found that his hearing had diminished somewhat and he was diagnosed as suffering from Menière's disease. Jonathan was given a drug called Stemetil (generic name prochlorperazine), which greatly eased the dizzy spells but did nothing for the deafness or noises in his ears.

Jonathan eventually came to see me and I found that he had somewhat catarrhal membranes lining the outer ear and a large number of enlarged lymph nodes on both sides of his neck. I treated him with ultrasonic waves, massage and electrical treatment to reestablish good drainage from his ears. Jonathan's trouble slowly cleared, and after 17 treatments he was more or less free of the noises and had no more dizzy spells.

The orthodox treatment for Menière's disease is largely symptomatic: drugs to damp down the dizzy spells when they come and, in extreme cases, an operation to destroy the inner ear when the dizzy spells become unbearable.

Vestibulitis

The vestibule is a cavity in the inner ear and part of the semi-circular canal complex. It contains sensitive hairs in its walls and a stone or stones which are pulled by gravity to the bottom of the cavity. These give a very sensitive interpretation of any slight change in the positioning of the body. Vestibulitis is an inflammation of the lining of the vestibule and a common cause of dizziness. It is often associated with a cold, but can come on without any other disease being present. Treat as for other ear problems (see page 215).

    See also chapter 6.

ECZEMA

It comes as a surprise to many people to discover that eczema is often triggered by a throat infection caused by the streptococcal bacteria. This particular strain of bacteria puts out a toxin which weakens the defence system in the throat, but also gets into the bloodstream. Once it has entered our circulation it has the capacity to affect any tissue similar to the throat membrane – including the skin and the membranes lining the joints. This explains the common and surprising origin of eczema and aching joints (*see* Joint Pain below) and why the two conditions often occur together.

When the skin is disturbed by this toxin it can cause a red, often slightly raised, map-like rash, commonly on the neck and over the upper part of the chest. This is known as a 'strep' rash. A more common response is for the skin to become weakened and all its functions diminished, although, initially, there is no outward sign of this. It is only when patches of skin are subject to stress, such as irritation through rubbing movements across joints or exposure to cold air, that they erupt into the typical red scaly rash, usually scattered with spots, known as eczema (from the Greek meaning 'to boil over').

While damaged tonsils as a result of childhood infections are a common cause of eczema in adults, there may also be other factors involved. With babies and young children, however, a weakened lymph system is by far the most common reason.

If a child is overclothed – and therefore overheated – the throat, as we have already seen in chapter 4, is more prone to infection. The skin is also more likely to be moist, as the child secretes sweat in a desperate attempt to cool down. Combine this situation with the effect of the 'strep' toxin and you have two of the most common causes of infantile eczema. Allergies – especially food sensitivities – which increase the blood supply to the skin are also a common trigger.

The treatment of infantile eczema is very straightforward:

- reduce the child's clothes to a bare minimum
- ensure that she gets plenty of fresh air
- in all but extreme conditions, cut out the heating in the bedroom
- eliminate any foods that you suspect are causing sensitivities, especially cow's milk
- if the tonsils are damaged (see chapter 5 for guidelines), talk to your doctor about having them removed
- give regular massage to the lymph nodes in the neck area, particularly those in the lower part, near the collarbone (see page 218 for directions).

Alistair was just over two and a half when he came to see me. He had bad eczema on his elbows and at the back of his knees and thighs. It was also on the lower part of his stomach and behind his right ear. The rash looked very red and angry and had some nasty raw patches, especially in the creases of his knees.

Alistair had started having eczema fairly early in life, at about six months. At that stage it was mild and restricted to the area of skin behind his knees, and was only really visible when he caught a cold. It became much worse when he was weaned at nine months and, between the age of 18 months and two years, it had spread to those other areas that were involved when he first came to me. The eczema varied in appearance, but the crinkled, red map-like rash broken up by sore patches and little scabs were a constant feature.

On examination, the skin lesions were typical of infantile eczema. It was also very itchy and his mother found it very hard to stop him from scratching constantly. Alistair had enlarged lymph nodes in his groin and his armpits, his throat was rather red and his tonsils were very swollen and somewhat infected. The lymph nodes in his neck, extending down from the tonsil node under the angle of the jaw, were also swollen.

A large part of Alistair's problem seemed due to the state of his throat, which I attributed primarily to overclothing. I advised his mother to dress him as lightly as possible while still keeping him warm. I assured her that children of that age feel the cold a great deal less than adults think. I also recommended some treatment to the lymph nodes in his neck, groin and armpits which his mother could carry out at home. The other advice I gave her was to try and cut out cow's milk completely for a while to see if this made any difference.

When his mother brought Alistair back for a check-up, she reported that she had been massaging the lymph nodes as I had shown her and that he seemed a lot happier now that he was wearing much less clothing. The eczema had receded quite a bit and did not look so angry. Within a couple of months it had largely gone, except for patches on the backs of his knees. His mother went on treating him and we gave him some ultrasound on the remaining areas of eczema and on his throat, which eventually cleared up.

However, about a year later his mother brought him back as there had been a recurrence after a bad cold. It was almost certain that a streptococcal infection had invaded his throat and had 'devitalized' the skin, causing the eczema to break out. After treatment, the eczema again faded away, apart from a minor outbreak a few months after his mother reintroduced cow's milk. Alistair came off the milk and was fit again. About two years later he was able to tolerate cow's milk without any obvious problems.

EMPHYSEMA

Asthma causes a blockage of the breathing tubes – especially on exhaling – which raises the pressure of the air in minute air sacs called the alveoli, causing the sufferer to struggle for breath. This symptom (struggling for breath) is the outstanding feature of emphysema. Bronchitis blocks the smaller air passages in the lungs with similar results.

When the main breathing tubes are blocked, air can still get into the alveoli, but it may not be able to get out and the act of coughing puts so much pressure on the air-filled alveoli that it can actually blow them inside out. As more and more alveoli are affected, the lungs gradually lose their capacity to exchange oxygen and carbon dioxide.

At this stage the sufferer becomes what is known as a 'respiratory cripple' and, as a result of breathlessness, can often do little more than sit up and eat. The condition is generally considered to be irreversible because it is widely believed that the effects of emphysema are caused entirely by the blown-out alveoli and that, once this has happened, the tide cannot be turned.

However, according to my experience it is often the blockage of the little ducts leading to the alveoli which is a major cause of symptoms. Once you can unblock the tubes and open up access to the parts of the lung that are still capable of working, you will often find that a so-called 'respiratory cripple' can lead quite an active life. I have had several patients, like 68-year-old Martin, who have resumed a full range of activities once these lymph nodes have been treated and the tubes cleared.

Martin had been a heavy smoker, although he had given up six years before he first came to see me. He had also had one or two attacks of bronchial pneumonia and this had left him with a very limited breathing capacity, which meant he was no longer able to ride his horse, which he had loved doing. He became breathless just getting onto a horse, let alone actually riding one. He found walking very difficult as he lost his breath climbing even the gentlest slope. He was diagnosed as having emphysema and was told that nothing could be done except to give him a little physiotherapy to improve his breathing.

I examined Martin and found that he had a number of swollen lymph nodes, especially at the base of his neck, above his collarbone. These are the ones that drain the upper part of the lung and the bronchial tree. He also had spasm of the muscles in the thoracic spine with resulting swelling of the tissues in that area. An x-ray showed that he had a number of enlarged lymph nodes in the area around the root of the lung.

Martin was treated with massage and ultrasonic waves to the lymph nodes in his neck and with electrical treatment to the mid-thoracic muscles. He was also given ultrasonic treatment to the lymph nodes in that area.

Martin's condition improved dramatically as the fluid drained out of the membranes lining the millions of tiny branches of the breathing tubes that lead to the alveoli. This opened up many alveoli that were still functional but had been bypassed because the tubes leading to them had been blocked. Martin's breathing was so much better that he was able to go riding again.

Four years later he had another attack of bronchitis following a bout of flu and this had left him a bit breathless. With his past history he was very worried about this, so he came to see me straight away. However, after only four treatments he was back on his horse again. That was six years ago and I haven't seen him again, but I have had a number of patients from the area who report that Martin is still riding and remains reasonably fit and well.

See also Asthma, Bronchitis, Hay Fever.

EPILEPSY

Epilepsy is usually caused by a permanent lesion, or scar, in the brain. Every so often this triggers a shower of impulses which fire all over the brain, sending it into a state of uncontrolled activity. This is manifested as an epileptic fit. The scar has the effect of slightly altering the brainwaves. This is clearly visible when an EEG – an electrical charting of the brain – is taken.

When a fit is in progress, the whole brain function is totally disorganized, but there is no explanation as to why the fit takes place at one particular time, leaving the brain working normally the rest of the time. Drugs which damp the brain down can be very effective in controlling the fits, although they have other, less desirable, side-effects. Once started, these drugs often have to be taken for life.

My theory offers a basis for a treatment that can, in many cases, control the initiation of a fit without resorting to drugs, although a (greatly reduced) dosage is sometimes still needed. It has often been noted that attacks of epilepsy occur with a cold, a sore throat or any conditions that precipitate or aggravate an existing catarrhal condition. The reason is probably that, although the actual defect is present in the brain all the time, the triggering is brought about by congestion in the brain itself (*see* Cerebral Oedema).

The lymphatic drainage both of the brain and the throat goes through the lymph nodes in the neck. If the lymph nodes in the neck are swollen and have become obstructed through constant infections in the throat, they will cause the brain to become more congested whenever they themselves become overloaded. Sufferers often find that attacks cease completely or occur very infrequently after treatment to the lymph nodes in their neck.

A few years ago I sold my car to a dealer and, in the middle of all the negotiations, he suddenly mentioned that his seven-year-old daughter, Roseanne, had bad epileptic fits and asked whether I knew if anything could be done. He confessed he thought it was probably hopeless, but whenever he met a doctor he always asked the same question. It turned out that Roseanne had been having around 200 fits a year for several years. She had been to Great Ormond Street Hospital and was on a lot of drugs. He said that when she was heavily drugged the fits became less frequent, but she was not really enjoying life and the future looked bleak.

I suggested that he ask his doctor to refer Roseanne to me for a consultation. When she came, I discovered that she had had a lot of colds and sore throats throughout a large proportion of her life. On examination she turned out to have large, unhealthy, pus-filled tonsils. The tonsil nodes in the upper part of her neck were huge and a chain of enlarged lymph nodes led from these down to her collarbone.

I explained how these lymph nodes drain the brain and that it was possible, when she was delivered by forceps, that this might have damaged her brain very slightly. This might well create no problems in itself, but if the brain became very congested, causing impulses to short-circuit, it would be enough to give the child a fit.

When Roseanne had her tonsils removed, the surgeon said that they were some of the worst that he had seen. She made a good recovery from the operation and then had treatment to unblock the lymph nodes, mostly at home from her mother. She came for two sessions of electrical treatment to improve the drainage through the neck area, at the end of which her general health was transformed. After two or three weeks her doctor began to reduce the drugs until he was able to discontinue them completely. She has had no fits to the present day.

Not all epileptics will have such a good result as this, but the treatment almost always diminishes attacks and can eliminate them altogether.

EYE CONDITIONS

Blepharitis

Blepharitis is inflammation of the eyelid. When the tear duct becomes blocked, the tear fluid, having nowhere to go, dries on the skin, sometimes causing sores and ulcers to form around the eye. This condition weakens the eyelid and it may begin to turn outwards, triggering a further increase in secretions in an effort to keep the now exposed inner side of the eyelid moist – and further compounding the problem.

Roger, 62, found himself producing tears rather more readily than normal. Anything that upset his eyes, such as cold air or draughts, made the tears form. The problem grew steadily worse, so that the tears were overflowing his eyelids more or less all the time. As a result, he was getting sores around the drainage points and his lower eyelid was beginning to turn out a little. This problem had been going on for some two years when he came to me.

On examination, I found that the membranes of his eyes were very inflamed and the small duct in the corner of the eye had become blocked due to the swollen membranes lining both the eye and the duct. Roger also had a small amount of nasal catarrh and a large number of hard, enlarged lymph nodes on both sides of his neck.

We set about clearing the lymphatic channels running from the corner of his eyes, down over the cheek to the lymph nodes, and treated the lymph nodes themselves. The drainage started to improve. It was in fits and starts – he would be better for a short time and then the trouble would recur. However, gradually the trouble-free periods became longer until the condition was very much improved. Unfortunately he still had tears with cold winds and with colds and catarrh, but the loose eyelids returned to normal.

Blocked Tear Ducts

Any catarrhal condition affecting the membrane which lines the tear duct can result in a blockage. The result is that the tears are not able to take their usual exit route and instead continually spill out over the cheeks. This can become extremely uncomfortable in windy or cold weather.

The orthodox treatment is to prescribe drugs that will shrink the membrane and, if the condition becomes distressing, a glass tube may be inserted into the duct to ensure adequate drainage, or the duct can be surgically enlarged. However, this usually brings about only a temporary improvement as the natural reaction of the body to this surgical enlargement is to line the duct with fibrous tissue, which can easily block it off again at a later date.

The surest way to provide semi-permanent relief is using lymphatic treatment to improve the tissue drainage. This involves massaging from the inner corner of the eye, down across the cheekbone in the direction of the earlobe, moving down towards the angle of the jaw and the lymph nodes at the top of the neck. This needs to be followed by massage to the general lymph nodes in the neck. The treatment assists the lymph drainage from the lining of the tear duct and can do a great deal towards clearing any blockages. However, electrical treatment to the outer corner of the eye is often needed to restore proper drainage.

Cataracts

As we have already seen, the eye is a very complicated structure. Unlike the lens in a camera, the eye's lens has varying densities and can change its shape to enable it to focus the image on the retina. The lens is made up of living cells which depend on fluid filtering through them to keep them healthy. It requires a considerable amount of oxygen to keep the lens transparent, as so much energy is expended on this. If there is back-pressure caused by blockage of the lymph nodes, the filtration through the lens can become inadequate and the lens gradually turns opaque. This is known as a cataract.

People with cataracts start to notice that detail and colour diminish and the sun and light acquire a red-dominated glare – rather like the paintings of J M W Turner. At the end of his life, Turner had advanced cataracts and he painted what he saw.

The conventional treatment for cataracts is to wait until the visual defect is interfering with the individual's quality of life and then to remove the entire lens from its capsule. Nowadays it is substituted with an artificial lens, which is a very effective operation. Cataracts, however, can be helped in the early stages by improving the drainage away from the eye through the lymph nodes and making sure that the filtration away from the eye and nutritional supply to the eye are adequate. The treatment is the same as for other eye conditions (see 'Detachment of the Retina'). Ultrasonic waves directed at the eye itself can greatly accelerate the effect of the treatment.

Margaret, 69, was greatly troubled by two cataracts which she had had for around three years. She was a diabetic and, at that time, her ophthalmic surgeon was not keen to operate on her. She came to me to see if there was anything that could be done that did not involve surgery.

The membranes of her eyes were a little swollen, particularly at the point where the eyelids met. There was also a ridge of swelling on the white of her eye and she had a number of enlarged, hard lymph nodes in both sides of her neck. I decided that, if we could clear the blockages and make the drainage more efficient, this could be enough to improve the nutrition in her eyes and maintain the necessary supply of oxygen to keep the lens transparent.

She was given massage to her eyes and her lymph nodes, which were also treated with ultrasonic waves. At the same time Margaret had electrical treatment to stimulate the muscles around the eye to pump fluid back to the lymph nodes. She came for nine visits in all, by which time her eyes were altogether more comfortable and she no longer needed an operation. She did, however, have to come back several times a year for a number years to maintain the circulation to the eye.

The chance of successful treatment was high, as Margaret came to me at a fairly early stage. It is vital to catch the condition before it gets too advanced, as the lens begins to calcify after a time – and then the cataract becomes irreversible.

Conjunctivitis and Styes

If the conjunctival membrane lining the eye becomes devitalized due to minor blockages in the local lymphatic drainage, this lowers its resistance to infection and leads either to conjunctivitis (also called 'pink-eye') or to infections of the grease glands of the eyelashes, known as styes.

Conjunctivitis is an infection of the membrane, usually caused by a particular bacterium called Morax-axenfeld's bacillus, although other bacteria can be involved. The main symptom is a red, itchy eye and a feeling of grit – or glass – under the lid. A more severe attack causes crusts of dried mucus to form on the eyelashes, which can glue the eyelids together during the night, hence the term 'sticky eye', by which the condition is also known. Small children often have a degree of overall congestion in the area, which gives the bacillus the opportunity to infiltrate the tear glands, from where it can repeatedly reinfect the eye. Conjunctivitis may occur as a single acute outbreak or as part of an epidemic or as a recurring condition. It is highly contagious and is usually spread by hand-to-eye contact.

Alexander came to see me when he was 16. He was not a particularly robust young man and had suffered with a lot of colds in his early years, which he claimed to have grown out of by the age of seven. He had remained reasonably fit until he was about 12, when he had his first attack of conjunctivitis.

This was followed by another attack the following year, during which his eyelids became badly stuck together. The condition eventually improved with the application of suitable drops. However, the following year he developed a stye with mild irritation in his eye and, although this cleared with some ointment, further styes began to appear with worrying regularity.

At the time I saw him he had two styes on the same lid. On further examination, the membranes of both his eyes appeared red and slightly swollen. There was a chain of firm, enlarged lymph nodes in his neck, which ran from the top of his neck almost as far as his collarbone.

I gave Alexander some ointment to help get rid of the infection and electrical treatment to assist the muscles in pumping the fluid away from the membrane of his eye, down the lymphatic ducts towards the neck. He also had treatment with ultrasonic waves and massage to decongest the lymph nodes in his neck.

After nine treatments, Alexander's lymph nodes could hardly be felt. His eyes were still a little red and he still had one large stye, but this gradually cleared up. He developed two more styes over the next two years, but a little ointment cleared them fairly rapidly. After that, the problem seemed to fade and the membrane of his eye no longer looked so angry. He also commented that he felt a great deal better in himself and that his memory had improved and he was able to think more quickly – a common observation among people who have had their cervical nodes treated.

Single, acute attacks of both conjunctivitis and styes can usually be cured with the use of drops, ointments or, in extreme cases, an antibiotic. Styes can also be relieved by applying alternating hot and cold compresses for 30 seconds at a time. Recurrent attacks, which can be very troublesome, are almost always caused by lymphatic blockages, and treatment to the relevant nodes will usually help to bring the cycle to an end (see page 217 for massage instructions).

It is also important to boost levels of vitamins A, D and C to build up general resistance to infection. If either of these conditions persist, the overall health of the patient needs to be investigated as there may be some underlying problem, such as diabetes.

Detachment of the Retina

If the pressure at the back of the eye is reduced because of a deterioration in the tone of the muscles that move the eye and wrap around it (see diagram, page 89), the eye starts to 'grow' and lose its optimum roundness in order to restore tissue tension. This is because it is normal for all the cells in your body to press against each other, so they are accustomed to being constantly squeezed. If this pressure slackens off, then nature immediately sets about restoring it. For example, if you cut yourself, the exposed cells on one side of the wound start multiplying furiously until they join up with the ones growing in from the other side. When the cells meet in the middle, tissue tension is restored and the cell growth stops.

In the case of the eye, the lack of pressure on the back of the eyeball has a similar effect, causing the whole eye to enlarge. Since the retina is rigid and cannot enlarge, in bad cases it may separate and become detached from the inside of the eye. Detachment of the retina can happen with very bad short sight where the eyeball also increases in size. This is a serious matter which can lead to blindness.

It is vital to stress that, if a retinal detachment does occur, it requires the urgent attention of a skilled ophthalmic surgeon. However, additional treatment from a qualified physiotherapist to improve the drainage of lymph from the area and electrical treatment to stimulate the tone of the muscles can have a profound effect on the end result.

I have seen a number of cases where the retina was not attaching as well as could be expected. Treatment with ultrasonic waves to the eye itself and with surged faradism (see Part IV) to the corner of the eye, accompanied by massage from the eye down the lymph nodes in the neck, caused a fairly rapid improvement in the condition.

Arthur, aged 62, was coming to the end of a course of treatment to relieve severe pain on the left side of his chest, when he remarked that it was a great pity physical medicine could not help his eyes. He told me that he had had silicone injected into his left eye after a bad retinal detachment, which was designed to press the retina against the back of the eye in the hope that it might re-attach.

The months passed by, but unfortunately the retina showed no sign of refixing to the eyeball. I told him that, as long as his surgeon agreed, I could give him treatment which would both bring the eyeball closer to the retina and greatly improve the repair mechanism in the eye. His surgeon agreed, so he was given massage to improve the lymph drainage from the eye as well as to the lymph nodes in his neck. He was also treated with ultrasonic waves in three-minute bursts to the eyeball itself. In three weeks the surgeon noticed a marked improvement and, in two more months, he was able to take out the silicone in Arthur's eye, leaving the retina firmly in place.

Provided that the condition is not too advanced and the eyeball has not grown excessively, it is possible to restore normal sight or, at least, prevent any further deterioration. Patients with retinal detachments must be managed by an ophthalmic consultant as the mainstay of their treatment, and any other treatment given only with their permission.

Glaucoma

This condition occurs when there is a dramatic rise in the finely balanced pressure of the fluid within the eye, which has the effect of compressing and obstructing the blood vessels which nourish the optic nerve. The early symptoms of glaucoma are headaches and seeing rings around artificial lights when looking at them. If the pressure suddenly rises to a dangerous level, the headache becomes severe and the patient feels ill.

It is sometimes caused by a shift in the angle between the cornea and the back part of the focusing chamber, which can block the exit hole of the 'drains' (see diagram, page 89), leading to a build-up of pressure in the fluid in the anterior chamber of the eye. This puts extra strain on the whole of the eye, distorting the shape of the cornea and further diminishing the filtration angle.

Abdul suffered from many symptoms, including seeing rings around lights. After an eye test, it was established that he was suffering from mild glaucoma. Preferring to avoid surgery if possible, he came to see me. I examined him and found that he had a large number of enlarged hard lymph nodes in the upper part of the neck and a history of sore throats at a young age. These sore throats continued until he was about 19, when he had finally had his tonsils out.

Although Abdul had made a good recovery from the operation, the lymph nodes draining the tonsils remained very enlarged, as did those on either side of his neck. I treated these and gave him electrical treatment to the muscles around his eyes and face, to pump away excess fluid from the eyes down to the lymph nodes. Abdul had 17 treatments in all, at the end of which the pressure had virtually returned to normal. He came back the following year for three more visits. After three years, the pressure was completely normal and he had no further trouble.

If you can improve the drainage and help the fluid in the ducts to drain away satisfactorily, then, in early cases, the pressure will automatically drop to a normal level. The treatment, which involves giving surged faradism to the corner of the eye and massage from the eye across the cheekbone to the ear and all the lymph glands in the neck, has been of immense help to a large number of people.

It is important to treat the problem in the early stages because if the pressure is allowed to continue for any length of time it will permanently damage the retina, leading to blindness. However, it cannot be stressed too strongly that professional advice from an ophthalmologist must always be sought and followed.

Short Sight

The movements of the eye depend on muscles which wrap around it and pull it to look at whatever you want to see. Like all muscles in the body, these have 'tone' – a steady and continuous contraction which increases when the muscle is required to work. With perfect eyesight, the tone of these muscles squeezes the back of the eye slightly forwards so that the image falls on the retina exactly in focus. If the muscles lose some of their tone, the eyeball elongates and, according to the laws of physics, will only be able to focus on close objects and not see clearly in the distance (see diagram, page 89). With short sight, the eyeball tends to be too long from front to back. As the retina is now optically in the wrong place, the lens can no longer focus on distant objects, although near things can be seen even closer up.

In younger people, the group of muscles which controls the focusing works harder than any other part of the eye. If the lymphatic drainage from the eye is impaired, then it is difficult for these muscles to relax after contracting for a period of time, for example, after reading. To offer an analogy: if you keep your fist clenched for several minutes, you will find that your fingers are stiff when you try to open your hand and you may find it hard to straighten them out completely. In terms of the eye, this lack of flexibility interferes with your ability to see a distant object, which means you will be classified as short-sighted and given glasses to bring distant objects closer.

In my view, wearing glasses to correct short sight can exaggerate the problem. Because your vision is directed through the optical centre of the lens, it restricts the movement of the eye. This means that the outside muscles become slack with disuse and so exert even less pressure on the back of the eye, causing the eyeball to lengthen further, which increases the focusing defect. I would recommend the weakest possible prescription and advise restricting the use of glasses to when absolutely necessary. Contact lenses, by contrast, strengthen the lens of the eye by allowing full movement and enabling the lens to make its own accommodation.

Once short sight has been diagnosed, many people spend the rest of their lives behind a pair of lenses. However it is worth questioning this approach, as lymphatic drainage treatment may be able to help.

One patient who stands out in my mind is Hank, a 17-year-old American boy who came to see me some years ago. His father was very high up in the American Air Force and Hank had every intention of following in his father's footsteps and becoming a pilot. Unfortunately, he was found to be short-sighted and, at that time, there was no chance of him becoming a pilot without perfect vision.

On examination, Hank had enlarged hard lymph nodes in both sides of his neck, and the membranes of his eyes were slightly swollen. I decided that this was why the focusing muscles were not working properly – partly because of the poor circulation to these muscles and partly because of congestion surrounding the nerve centres which help control the focusing. Hank received treatment to the lymph nodes in his neck and electrical stimulation to the muscles around his eye, which was intended to pump the fluid away from the eye back to these lymph nodes. He was also given massage around the eyes down in the direction of the lymph nodes in the neck.

After 11 treatments, Hank's vision had become normal again and he wrote to me about four months later saying that he had passed his medical test and was able to take up the career as a pilot he had so desperately wanted.

An improvement in general health can also help the sight. Exercises designed to get the eye to focus on objects at increasing distances can be of some value, but they will only produce an improvement as long as you continue to do them.

Squints

One reason why people squint is because one of the muscles that moves the eye is either weak or too short, so the direction of the vision of the two eyes is different. In this situation, surgical correction to straighten up the affected eye is required. A more common reason, though, is that one eye focuses better than the other, and, because the brain refuses to accept a picture degraded by the poorly focused image, it pushes the bad eye to one side and suppresses its image in favour of the unadulterated picture from the other. There is nothing wrong with the muscles that control movement of the eye.

A primary cause of an imbalance of this kind is a partial blockage of the cervical lymph nodes which drain the eye (see diagram, page 82). If these nodes are not functioning properly and the drainage is poor, it will affect the muscles wrapped around the eye and also those used for focusing, causing the eye to be short sighted.

The lymphatic treatment is the same as for short sight, concentrating on the weaker eye, and it may be necessary to put a patch over the stronger eye for an hour or two every day to get the brain to start using the weaker eye again. Up to the age of six or seven, exercises with a piece of equipment called a stereoscope can be helpful in restoring binocular vision. If the lymphatic drainage can be improved and the vision in both eyes restored to normal, the squint should disappear. However, the brain may need to be convinced by exercises that it is now possible to join the images from both the eyes.

It is important to stress that, the younger a person is treated, the better the results are likely to be. It may be possible to restore stereo-scopic – or 3D – vision up to the age of six, and binocular vision – where the picture from both eyes is joined to make a single picture but without any depth to it – up to 12 years. After this age it becomes difficult to achieve even binocular vision with my treatment, although it does, very rarely, get extraordinary results, as Naomi's case shows.

Naomi was 23 when she was brought to see me by her father. She had a very bad convergent squint and had already had two operations to straighten her eyes. These had been successful for a time, but then her eyes had starting squinting again. Both eyes were independently capable of a full range of movement and I decided that the squint was due to the differ-ence of the focusing ability of the two eyes. In other words, the eye that was not properly in focus was degrading the image of the other eye and the brain had decided to dispense with that eye and push it out to one side.

I explained to Naomi and her father that, given her age, it was highly unlikely that any treatment would be successful. However, her father said that as long as there was the slightest chance it was worth trying. So I start-ed treating Naomi and, to my amazement, after the fourth visit she said that her eyes had briefly come together in the morning.

As the treatment went on, Naomi's eyes continued to come together for longer periods in the morning. However, as soon as she got tired they wandered off again. After 18 visits, her eyes were together most of the time, except when she got excited or tired or if she was suffering from a cold. As the years went by, the cohesion of the two eyes into forming a single picture became stronger and stronger until eventually Naomi stopped squinting altogether.

The reason why it is much easier to correct squints at a young age can be explained by a basic difference between human and animal babies. Most animals, when they are born, have a great deal of pre-programming in their brains, whereas human babies are born with only the most basic mechanisms, such as sucking and breathing, built in. All the rest has to be learned. The advantage of this is that we can learn a behavioural pattern for just about any circumstances or conditions in which we find ourselves. The penalty, however, is that we are the most helpless babies in the animal world.

At birth, your brain is a huge pad of blotting paper waiting to absorb information. When it is empty, the brain is able to deal with the most complicated things. As it gathers more and more information, it has less space to allocate to intricate manoeuvres. At each stage of your life, there comes a point when you are actually too old to perform a particular function if you have not learned it already. Stereoscopic vision is a feat that has to be learned early in life and can be acquired only with difficulty after the age of six.

See also chapter 6.

FOOD SENSITIVITIES

Food sensitivities are a sort of allergy. In a true allergy the symptoms come on almost as soon as the food is eaten, usually in the form of a skin rash or breathing difficulties. With food sensitivities, the reaction occurs more slowly and lasts for a period of approximately five days. For this reason it is not always obvious which food is causing the trouble. To further cloud the picture, when the offending food is eaten it tends to cause an outpouring of cortisol from the adrenal glands, which gives the patient a feeling of immense well-being. As a result, they often develop a craving for the food and come to regard it as a guaranteed pick-me-up, rather than identifying it as the cause of their problems.

The most common culprits are cow's milk and its by-products, white flour, gluten, coffee, yeast, sugar and tomatoes.

Wheat is one of the most common causes of food sensitivity in all age groups. The main symptom is usually tiredness, but indigestion and irritable bowel syndrome, respiratory obstruction, snoring, acne or spots on the skin can also occur.

GASTRITIS

see chapter 5

GLANDULAR FEVER

Glandular fever affects the lymph nodes throughout the body. Gentle massage of the main groups and a massive intake of vitamin B to replace the destruction brought about by the virus helps the patient to get over the disease more quickly and makes a relapse much less likely. Sufferers also benefit from taking trace elements such as magnesium and iron.

GLAUCOMA

see Eye Conditions

GLUE EAR

see Ear Problems

HAY FEVER

For many people the summer months are marred by hay fever. The greatest sympathy must go to sufferers sitting exams, as the authorities could not have chosen a worse moment in the year for them.

It is called 'hay fever' because the first substance found to cause it was hay pollen, and the symptoms are almost identical to those of a classic fever or cold:

- a streaming – and blocked – nose
- swollen and irritated eyes
- feverishness
- a general feeling of being unwell.

The mind also becomes affected, with poor recall and concentration as well as a degree of irritability. The difference between hay fever and a cold is that a cold virus is eliminated in a few days, after which the person regains normal health. With hay fever, on the other hand, the poor victim suffers as long as the affecting substances remain present in the air.

Hay fever is almost always a sensitivity or allergy of the membranes that line the nose and nasal sinuses, which have become swollen and excessively irritable because the lymph nodes draining them are partially obstructed.

When pollens land and adhere to sticky membranes, they aggravate the inflammation, causing an increase in the circulation at that particular point. Unfortunately, because the body is intent on warding off invaders at all costs, it goes into overdrive, triggering a reaction – to that one speck of pollen – worthy of an invasion on a massive scale. This is known as an allergic response. An allergy is a normal response of the body to an irritant taken to an abnormal intensity.

So, an inhaled particle of a generally harmless substance can send the nose, sinuses, throat and eyes all into an advanced state of inflammation in the body's misguided attempt to expel an invader that never arrives. Sadly, this 'protection' causes greater distress to the sufferer than the invader would have done.

Around 30 years ago I would have said with some confidence that it was possible to relieve almost every case of hay fever by getting rid of any low-grade infection in the nose, sinuses and throat. These days, however, there is such a high level of irritation present in the air from pollution and the proliferation of pollens coming from grass, the ever-increasing number of municipal flowering trees and shrubs, and certain crops (especially oil seed rape), that treating the infection is seldom sufficient.

Conventional treatment for hay fever is with anti-allergy pills, decongesting sprays, cortisone sprays and, in extreme cases, long-acting cortisone injections. These injections tend to be extremely effective in people with a short hay fever season, as the benefits last for at least three weeks and they have virtually no side-effects. However, my treatment offers complete relief for some sufferers, and a considerable reduction in the medication needed for others.

The prescription is the same as for sinus trouble. The sinuses and cheekbones need to be massaged and the lymph drained in the direction of the lymph nodes in the neck. Ultrasonic waves and electrical treatment to these areas is also recommended (see Part IV).

HEARING DIFFICULTIES

see Ear Problems

INFERTILITY PROBLEMS

see Salpingitis

INNER EAR CONDITIONS

see Ear Problems

IONIZATION

The particles in the air can either be positively or negatively charged. If there is movement in the air, generated for instance by winds, air conditioning, fan heaters or car heaters, the air particles become positively charged.

The body scarcely reacts to negatively charged particles. However, the platelets in the blood react to positively charged particles, as these are absorbed through the lung with the oxygen and secrete a substance called serotonin, which aggravates any inflammatory condition present in the body. This explains why, when elderly ladies say 'their rheumatics are cruel', it is often an indication that the weather is going to change (see page 39).

IRRITABLE BOWEL SYNDROME

Probably one of the most common causes of this condition is sensitivity to foodstuffs such as white flour, gluten, cow's milk and coffee.

However, it may also occur when the sympathetic ganglia in the chest area malfunction, causing an excess of acid in the stomach and excessive peristalsis (the 'pumping effect' of the muscles of the bowel), causing diarrhoea.

The symptoms associated with irritable bowel syndrome are very similar to some of those produced by chronic appendicitis.

When food sensitivities develop, the lining of the stomach and/or bowel becomes inflamed and forms a kind of low-grade allergy to certain foods. The main effect of this is constitutional, causing symptoms such as tiredness, hyperactivity and depression, which do not seem to be related to any abdominal problem.

In many cases, however, abdominal symptoms are the feature that the sufferer notices. When any poison or infection invades the bowel, its main weapon is to remove it by vigorous action, leading to diarrhoea. This creates the additional problem of undigested food being hurried into the large bowel, where it ferments, producing toxins that further irritate the bowel. In this way, a long-lasting condition is set up.

Treatment is divided into several categories:

- The stomach is almost always inflamed in this condition. The superior splanchnic ganglion, a 'computer' that lives on the muscles of the thoracic spine, under normal conditions switches the acid of the stomach off. When it malfunctions, this control is upset and acid continuously pours into the stomach, inflaming the membrane that lines it. This can be corrected with lymphatic drainage treatment to the mid-thoracic region.

- Food sensitivities need to be pinpointed as far as possible, so that the culprits may be removed from the diet long enough to allow the sufferer to recover. They can normally be cautiously reintroduced after the patient has been free of symptoms for about a year. The continuous diarrhoea needs to be controlled by drugs that damp down the over-activity of the bowel muscles. There are several medications that will achieve this result, but I have found that Lomotil (generic name diphenoxylate) is much the most effective.

■ The lymph nodes draining the bowel, where accessible, should be treated with massage. Those located deeper in the abdomen can be treated with (longwave) ultrasound. The blockage of these nodes results in a catarrhal condition of the bowel lining, which also contributes to the diarrhoea.

JOINT PAIN

We have already seen how the toxins which are put out by bacteria to devitalize the lining of the throat can also affect the similar membrane lining the joints (*see* Eczema). Cynthia's case is a useful illustration of this.

Cynthia came to see me at the age of 31. She was not feeling at all well in herself. She tired easily and her brain felt, in her words, 'woolly'. Her other worry was that she was beginning to get pains in some of her joints. Her left knee had started aching about three months before and it was very uncomfortable, especially when going downstairs. Cynthia had been fully investigated, but the doctors had found nothing wrong. She said that two of the fingers in her left hand and the digit finger of the right hand were a little swollen and painful. She also had a slight ache in her left hip at times.

When I asked about sore throats, Cynthia looked a bit perplexed, because she could not see any obvious connection. However, she told me that she had started having occasional sore throats when she was very young and these had increased in frequency until she was 18, when her health had shown an overall improvement. By the time I saw her, the sore throats were only sporadic and usually triggered by a cold.

On examining her, I could not find much wrong with her actual joints. Although they were swollen and slightly tender, they all had full movement and her blood count was normal. However, her tonsils were large and very unhealthy – as were the associated lymph nodes – and a number of others could be felt on both sides of her neck. It seemed to me that her tonsils were damaged, and I asked an ear, nose and throat surgeon to look at her. He agreed with my diagnosis and took out her tonsils, which were apparently in a very bad state indeed.

Once her system had had time to recover from the operation, Cynthia felt much more lively and considerably less tired. Best of all, the problems with her joints disappeared.

LARYNGITIS

Laryngitis is an inflammation of the larynx, or voice-box. My patients include a variety of professional voice-users, such as actors and singers, whose careers depend on the quality of their voices. If they suffer from intermittent voice loss or hoarseness it affects both their reputation and their livelihood. Thankfully, I have been successful in treating many of them, thus restoring and – in some cases – even improving their voices.

Our vocal cords have to be shiny and dry in order to vibrate effectively. If they become abnormally damp, they do not work so well. When we use our voice it involves a large muscular effort to tighten the vocal cords sufficiently to make them vibrate at different pitches. The greater the muscular effort, the greater the amount of blood needed in that area. It follows, then, that a fairly large quantity of fluid has to drain away from the larynx when it is involved in the considerable effort of projecting the voice while singing or acting.

If the cervical lymph nodes are congested, this fluid cannot drain away, causing back-pressure and a serious waterlogging of the vocal cords, which impairs their ability to vibrate. The first sign of this is squeakiness, which then turns into mild hoarseness and culminates in varying degrees of voice loss.

A single attack of laryngitis is not an ailment which people usually take to their doctor. It is when someone perpetually loses his voice that problems arise, especially if his career prospects or livelihood is threatened. The usual treatment is a throat spray either of an antibiotic or an adrenalin-like substance to dry up the throat, often combined with an anti-allergy drug – or a combination of all three.

In sharper infections, the antibiotic would be given in capsule form. However, this is not a satisfactory form of treatment for recurrent attacks, because the sufferer does not form antibodies against the infection. The drying-up drugs cut back the circulation, only to be followed by a massive surge of blood to make up for the temporary drought. This in itself can lead to loss of voice and certainly reduces resistance to subsequent infections.

In the case of an emergency with a performer, I sometimes recommend using a cortisone spray to the larynx and an antibiotic to get through a performance. A cold spray on the larynx – for just 30 seconds or so – also helps to decongest it and will offer temporary relief. However, for more permanent relief it is necessary to treat the overburdened lymph nodes above the collarbone and around the larynx itself with massage and ultrasonic waves.

LEG ULCER

see Ulcers

MEMBRANES

Membranes line most of your mouth, nose, bronchial tree and intestinal tract. They are generally made up of what are known as 'pavement' cells which are large, flat and very thin. This means that the blood supply with its protective substances is very close to the surface and can deal quickly and easily with any infection or injury. When lymphatic drainage is poor, the pavement cells try to bolster their defence by piling up on top of each other. Unfortunately this has the opposite effect, because the thicker the membranes get, sometimes reaching many thousand times their original depth, the further removed the surface cells are from the blood supply and defence mechanism. Bacteria are therefore able to invade the membrane and survive.

For this reason, thickened membranes greatly lower your resistance to infection as well as making it more difficult to throw infection off. Mucus is secreted by glands in the membranes to wash away any 'bugs' or foreign bodies. Membranes do contain some basic antibodies but, as the invasion continues, further protection against invaders comes from the lymph system through the blood. One of the greatest benefits of improved lymphatic drainage is that, as the membranes shrink back to their normal size, full defensive service is restored.

When a membrane is swollen it becomes sticky and the little hairs on the surface, which normally move in organized waves to sweep away foreign bodies, become completely engulfed in the swelling and no longer do their job. Irritating particles are therefore able to land

and fix on the membrane, inflaming it and aggravating the existing congestion. At the same time, secretions from the membrane flow out, causing a discharge.

MENIÈRE'S DISEASE

see Ear Problems

MENSTRUAL PROBLEMS

see Painful Periods

MIDDLE EAR INFECTION

see Ear Problems

MINERALS AND TRACE ELEMENTS

Up to the teenage years, children's digestion and absorption of minerals and trace element substances is generally good enough not to require supplementation. Even in a somewhat limited diet there are usually enough trace elements to maintain good health. With stomach upsets, however, absorption may be affected and deficiencies may therefore arise.

Magnesium is one of the minerals that the body requires in larger quantities. Among its many important functions, magnesium is used by red cells to activate the haemoglobin's ability to carry oxygen. If the magnesium level in the body is low, a person may feel tired and 'woolly' in the head. Magnesium is not an easy substance to administer, but it can be injected (very painfully!). It is often utilized better if taken orally in various forms. One of the best formulations is Magnesium OK, where it is combined with many other trace elements.

Trace elements, although they are only needed by the body in small quantities – it is definitely advisable to stick to the RDA – are nevertheless essential to health. They include iron, chromium, copper, iodine, manganese, selenium, silicon, sulphur and zinc. Zinc and magnesium cream can be used on boils and badly healing wounds to draw the fluid out and improve tissue circulation.

See also chapter 4.

MULTIPLE SCLEROSIS

This is a disease where the connective tissue of the spinal cord becomes inflamed and fluid accumulates around it. The fluid presses on the nerves and, as a result, can interfere with their conduction. In the early stages, once the infection has subsided the fluid will slowly be absorbed and the nerves able to recover their function, unless they have been permanently damaged. As the disease progresses, however, the fluid remains, the symptoms become more constant and the damage to the nerves more extensive and permanent.

If the fluid can be encouraged to drain away more rapidly, the attacks become shorter and considerably less intense and the damage is limited; in addition, the general state of the sufferer is improved. Since it is a condition which involves the back as much as the lymphatic system, massage, electrical and ultrasonic treatment to the spinal muscles can make all the difference.

NAUSEA

This can be general or specific. Many children develop certain symptoms at the beginning of an illness – it may be a stomach ache, a headache or feeling nauseous. So that particular child, whatever illness is about to befall her, will often feel sick as one of the preliminary warning signs. Among the specific causes of nausea, the most common is eating unsuitable food; the next most common is intestinal infection. There are a number of rarer diseases which also cause sickness or vomiting. If there is no obvious cause, then medical help should be sought.

NIGHTMARES

In my experience, nightmares can have physical causes including a respiratory obstruction linked to snoring, or problems with the tonsils. Since the soft palate becomes floppy when it is waterlogged, treatment to the lymph nodes which drain it will tighten it up so that it no longer causes an obstruction. The tonsils may be enlarged as a result of an immediate infection or because they are damaged and permanently swollen. Damage to the tonsils can also cause the adenoids to undergo considerable compensatory enlargement. If so, the tonsils should be removed (see chapter 5).

OSTEOMYELITIS

Osteomyelitis is an infection of the bone marrow which can be very difficult to throw off because:

- The infection is surrounded by inert bone so there is no defence mechanism that can easily deal with the problem.
- The circulation to some of the bone is patchy and may well be only at one end of the infection which is effectively in a 'tube'.
- The bone itself acts as a refuge for some of the bacteria.

The healing and repair process can be hugely accelerated by lymphatic drainage techniques in the area. Even chronic conditions can be stimulated into a complete recovery.

PAINFUL PERIODS

If the lymphatic drainage from the uterus becomes obstructed, then the muscles of the uterus wall and its lining membrane are likely to become waterlogged. Under these conditions, the blood thickens slightly and may clot. Consequently, it tends to be pushed out with more difficulty than usual during menstruation. As the cavity of the uterus is quite small, it has difficulty expelling these clots and goes into intense contractions (which cause the pain) in order to get rid of them.

The usual treatment for painful periods is painkillers and anti-spasmodic drugs to stop the cramps. However, these offer only temporary relief. If other readily diagnosable causes have been eliminated, my treatment may provide a permanent answer by reducing the congestion in the area and preventing the formation of clots so that normal contractions are sufficient to do the job.

The treatment is virtually the same as for cystitis (see page 221). The only difference is that there may be a problem in the lumbar region which also needs treating. Symptoms of painful periods may take some time to subside. This is because the body is so quick to form a habit that, even though the conditions are improved, it is slow to realize that there is no need to produce a cramp to expel the fluid.

Selina was 23 and she came to me with a painful back. She had a great deal of spasm in the muscles on either side of her spine, which we treated. Just before one visit she cancelled her appointment because she was having such a painful period that she had to retire to bed. When she came back for the next treatment, I suggested that I have a look as I might be able to help this problem, too.

On examination I discovered that Selina had enlarged abdominal lymph nodes, so these were treated at the same time as her back.

At her three-month check-up, Selina reported that her periods had been lighter and much less painful, although the treatment had made them heavier initially. At her six-month check-up, she said that although her periods were still uncomfortable, this could now be relieved by normal painkillers.

There is little doubt that Selina's bad back also played a part in her painful periods, because the lower section of the lumbar spine sends out nerves that go to the uterus and control the blood vessels and muscles there. If these nerves are disturbed by back trouble, this can also be a cause of painful periods.

Congestion in this area can also prevent women from becoming pregnant, as it stops the fertilized ovum from implanting securely onto the wall of the uterus. Treatment to reduce the swelling can sometimes resolve the problem.

PERITONITIS

The peritoneum is a bag that lines the abdominal cavity. The inner side covers all the abdominal organs, including the bowel, and is moulded to their shape. The outer layer covers the entire wall of the abdominal cavity. An infection of the peritoneum is a serious matter as it does not possess a particularly strong defence mechanism. A child with chronic appendicitis feels pain where the shared nerve comes out between the ribs and the tummy button. If, however, the infection breaks through the wall of the appendix and goes as far as the peritoneal membrane lining the outside of the appendix, the pain can immediately be accurately located as it shifts to the actual site of the trouble in the right lower quarter of the abdomen. This is a very serious warning and emergency medical help is required.

See also Appendicitis.

PINK EYE

see Eye Conditions – Conjunctivitis

POLYPS

These generally occur – in either the bladder or the sinuses – only if the membranes lining them are swollen. A normal membrane should be like marble tiles – flat, smooth and shiny. If the membrane becomes waterlogged, it may start to grow into little heaps. The body regards these heaps as foreign bodies and tries to get rid of them by sucking them off. As a result, they lengthen and develop into a large blob at the end of a thin stalk, which we call a polyp.

Polyps may come about as a result of infection, but more commonly they occur for no reason.

For polyps caused by an infection, treatment to the lymph nodes in the groin and the neck respectively will help polyps in the bladder or sinuses (see page 221), although the infection needs to be addressed at the same time.

Polyps that come about for no obvious reason do not respond to this treatment. If they have to be removed by snaring, effective lymph drainage will often prevent polyps from reforming. When a polyp in the bladder breaks off, its blood supply leaks and the patient passes blood.

POSITIVE IONIZATION

see Ionization

PSYCHOLOGICAL PROBLEMS

There are well-recognized psychological problems associated with childhood, but the connection is seldom made between persistent throat infections or trouble with the tonsils and a deterioration in a child's behaviour. Since the lymph nodes in the neck drain the brain as well as the throat, sinuses and ears, any obstruction causes the brain to become mildly waterlogged. Children suffering from this mild form of cerebral oedema have poor concentration and a poor short-term memory. They also react very badly to discipline or authority. This sort of child is a teacher's nightmare and tends to get pushed to the back of the class, where the trouble intensifies. Simple lymphatic drainage treatment to the lymph nodes in the neck, and – if damaged – the removal of the tonsils, makes a spectacular difference.

See also Cerebral Oedema.

RETINA, DETACHMENT OF

see Eye Conditions

RHEUMATOID ARTHRITIS

A type of arthritis in which the joints of the body become painful, swollen, stiff and often deformed. This is accompanied by mild fever and fatigue. It usually strikes in early adulthood, and, in the patients I have seen, is virtually always associated with infected and damaged tonsils.

Sufferers tend to have a history of constant sore throats up to the age of seven or eight, followed by a 'well' phase lasting about 10 years. Then, around the age of 17, they develop a sore throat and hot, painful joints and their tonsils flare up. This is one of the auto-immune system's many malfunctions. What seems to happen is that the lymph nodes start to produce slightly faulty antibodies to a toxin put out by a chronic streptococcal infection and the patient becomes allergic to this antibody, which causes inflammation of the joints. It is my belief that if damaged tonsils were removed in childhood, the condition would be far less likely to occur.

Emma, aged 27, was my secretary. She had been a little prone to throat trouble, but it was not so bad that it interfered with her job. Then one day she asked me if I would look at her wrist because she thought that she must have sprained it, although she had no memory of doing so. She showed me a hot, painful, rather swollen wrist. I then looked at her other joints and found she also had a swollen and tender ankle and several swollen fingers.

I asked if she had a sore throat at the time and she said she had had one for about three days. Her tonsils were heavily infected. A blood test came up positive for toxins which can affect the joints; a culture of the bacteria showed it to be strep viridans. I insisted that she should be rushed to hospital to have her tonsils removed immediately.

All of Emma's joints flared up directly after the operation and she was in a great deal of pain, but this settled down in a few weeks. Over the next couple of years she did still experience a slight pain in her wrist from time to time, but the trouble gradually faded out. I am quite sure that, if Emma's tonsils had been left in for many more months, the condition would suddenly have developed into full-blown rheumatoid arthritis. It would, most likely, by then have been too late to do anything. Taking her tonsils out at that stage would not have cured the trouble because, by then, Emma would have developed an allergy to the toxins and the most minute infection present in her throat would have been enough to maintain the arthritis.

SALPINGITIS

Abdominal congestion can result in infections of the vagina, cervix or uterus spreading as far as the Fallopian tubes. This leads to a condition called salpingitis, when the Fallopian tube becomes inflamed, which may prevent the ovum from passing into the uterus.

A friend, Elizabeth, who was about 27, suddenly announced that she was feeling 'rotten'. She started to shiver and had a real attack of the shakes. We took her temperature and found that it was quite high. She was beginning to get severe pains in her tummy and, after having a look at her, I was fairly certain that it was a gynaecological problem.

It was obviously an emergency, so I asked a gynaecologist friend of mine for his opinion. Elizabeth had been using an intra-uterine coil as a contraceptive and had recently had it removed. When the gynaecologist examined her, he discovered that she had a bad infection and there seemed to be a foreign body present. This turned out to be a second coil, which had become more or less impacted as the uterus had swollen around it. It had then become heavily infected.

The coil was removed under anaesthetic. However, when Elizabeth was told about it, she insisted that the coil had been removed the previous week. The true story then emerged: Elizabeth had gone to have the coil changed three years before at a clinic. Her notes said that the coil must have 'slipped out' at some time because they could not find it; another one was duly inserted. Meanwhile, the first coil had remained inside her for the entire three years.

This particular story seemed to have a happy ending. Elizabeth was put on antibiotics and made a good recovery. However, the time came when she wanted to become pregnant and, when after a time she remained unsuccessful, she decided to have a check-up.

The doctors found that Elizabeth's Fallopian tubes, which connect the ovaries to the uterus, were totally blocked. She was told that the gross infection caused by the coil was responsible and that there was no way that she would ever be able to have a baby naturally. One day when I was with her, she suddenly burst into floods of tears and told me this rather distressing tale.

I had a look at her and could feel a lot of firm adhesions in her abdomen. An x-ray showed shadows in the back part of the abdomen, behind the spinal cord, which looked like enlarged lymph nodes. She had treatment to these lymph nodes and ultrasound over her ovaries and uterus.

After 14 treatments and about five months later, Elizabeth announced that she was pregnant. The treatment to the lymph nodes had improved the drainage sufficiently to allow the white cells to dispose of most of the fibrous tissue and adhesions which had formed in order to seal off the infection. At the same time, the reduced congestion in the lining of her Fallopian tubes had created enough space to allow the ovum to pass from the abdominal cavity into the uterus. In due course Elizabeth gave birth to a healthy baby girl.

SCARLET FEVER

The true picture of scarlet fever, characterized by redness over a large area of the body and a very high temperature, is seldom seen. A modified version with 'strep' throat and a limited rash, say, on the chest, is relatively common. In almost all cases this is due to infected tonsils, which require removal.

SHINGLES

With shingles, the chicken pox virus attacks the connective tissue of the spinal cord, producing tremendous swelling which inflames and compresses the adjacent nerve tracks. This causes impulses to travel backwards along sensory nerves. The perceptors in the skin and local blood vessels are wrongly stimulated, causing a red rash and blisters along the line of the nerve. This is often mistakenly thought to be the actual site of the disease. If the nerves in the spinal cord are damaged, pain and/or numbness is felt. Once the body has destroyed the virus, in a few days the effects subside and, in many cases, disappear altogether.

Early treatment to reduce the build-up of fluid in the spinal cord around the inflamed area limits the severity of symptoms and speeds up recovery. This is achieved by massage, electrical and ultrasonic treatment to the muscles over the area involved.

SHORT SIGHT

see Eye Conditions

SINUSITIS

The less acute conditions affecting the sinuses are directly related to blockages of the cervical nodes (see diagram, page 82), which causes swelling of the membranes lining the sinuses.

Chronic sinusitis is a low-grade infection of the membrane. This is a more or less permanent state of affairs, but every so often there will be a marked flare-up in the condition – generally after a cold. This is often brought about by a blockage of the sinus opening, which prevents the fluid from draining away and so prolongs the infection.

Acute inflammation of the sinuses may occur in a completely healthy person who is momentarily overwhelmed by a virulent infection, and symptoms include headache, pain and usually a high fever. It is readily treated by antibiotics and, once brought under control, may not recur.

Many people who have trouble with their sinuses do not fully understand the role of these air-filled cavities within the body. Sinuses are air passages contained within the bones of your skull, which are mostly joined to the main airway inside the nose.

Your skull is there to protect your body's most delicate piece of equipment – your brain – and to act as a framework for the attachment of the very large muscles of your head. The bones of your skull have projections which provide a good fixing point for these powerful muscles, especially those used for chewing.

You would think, with all of these bony projections, that your skull would be too heavy for you to lift, but nature hollows the bones out, following the best engineering principles, and the resulting cavities are the sinuses. Of the 60 or so sinuses encapsulated within the body, the majority are small and insignificant, but a few of the large and more important ones have been given special names. The most troublesome are the maxillary, the frontal sinuses and the mastoid.

Like so many parts of the body, some of the sinuses double up their use. The inner and middle ear are actually built in a sinus, so problems of the middle ear and sinuses are often interrelated. In the same way that the Eustachian tube acts to equalize the air pressure inside and outside the middle ear, so the other sinuses have openings to the atmosphere to maintain a constant pressure inside and out.

If the membranes of the sinuses become swollen, then these openings can become blocked. The blood circulating in the lining membrane slowly absorbs the air in the sinus or middle ear, causing a vacuum. This is one of the causes of the painful symptoms of sinusitis. Of course the opposite effect can occur, when the blocked openings do now allow the fluid from a sub-acute or acute attack to drain away, so it is the increased pressure that causes the pain.

Liam, aged 67, came to see me about his catarrh and occasional headaches. He said that he had had trouble with his throat when he was small and had had his tonsils removed when he was 14. This operation improved his throat problems and general health very considerably.

However, when he was 27, Liam had a bad attack of flu, which was followed by bronchitis and some pain in the part of his head just above his eyebrows, particularly on the left side. This pain gradually cleared, but, about nine months later, Liam caught a cold and this was accompanied by heavy discharge from his nose. He started to experience severe pain in his forehead above his left eye and earache in his left ear.

Liam noticed that the catarrh subsequently increased and if, for example, he went out in cold weather or found himself in a very dusty atmosphere, the pain in his forehead became severe. As he got older, the catarrhal state steadily worsened. He had the septum of his nose (the partition which divided the two sides) examined and this turned out to be very bent to one side. So he had an operation to straighten it by removing some of its cartilage. This definitely improved his catarrhal condition by removing a partial obstruction to the frontal sinus duct, although the headache over his eye remained.

When I saw him, Liam had had two or three attacks of pain fairly close together. On one of these occasions, the pain was accompanied by a bad earache. He had been put onto antibiotics by his doctor; this helped to clear the problem temporarily, but it soon returned. He was given antibiotics again, but this time they had little or no effect.

On examination, Liam had a thick membrane lining his nose and there was some discharge dripping down the back of his throat from the nose and sinus area. The area over his left eyebrow was very tender. There were a large number of swollen, hard lymph nodes in both sides of his neck, especially the left side. The upper lymph nodes were tender to touch.

I decided that Liam's main problem was that these lymph nodes had become very congested. They were causing poor drainage from the membranes of the nose, particularly from the area at the top of the nose that includes the drainhole to the frontal sinus, which equalizes the pressure inside and outside the sinus and allows the fluid out. The swollen membrane was blocking the hole and, periodically, this caused a vacuum in the sinus which gave rise to a headache.

Liam had 14 treatments to unblock the lymph nodes and improve the lymph drainage from the area. After this, he was about 80 per cent better. When I saw him after three months he said his condition had improved considerably but it was still not quite right. It took a further six months before he was completely free of the sinusitis.

Patients suffering from sinusitis today are treated, as far as possible, with decongesting drugs, and if necessary, with antibiotics. They may also have the pus washed out of the sinus and then have it filled with an antibiotic. It is only in extreme cases that the patient is advised to have surgery. This is to enlarge the outlet and then strip out the membrane so it cannot swell and block the hole. Unfortunately, this means removing a wall that also keeps out the bacteria, so the sinus becomes more liable to infection. It is often said that once you have had your first operation on your sinuses, you will be a patient for the rest of your life – and it holds some truth.

To my mind, it makes far more sense to attempt to improve the natural lymphatic drainage. This allows the membranes to shrink so that air can pass in freely through the ducts and the problem is less likely to recur. Indeed, once the drainage is restored, the person actually acquires a very high resistance to infection. Many of my patients have boasted that they were sometimes the only member of their family to go through the winter without catching a cold.

The lymph nodes in the whole of the neck require treating; electrical treatment to the facial nerve is especially helpful (see page 212). It is also useful to check for any dental problems. If a tooth is projecting into the sinus or there is an infected root nearby, this can be a cause of trouble and needs to be dealt with.

When a person is suffering from sinusitis, the membranes of the maxillary sinus may become very swollen and eventually start to heap up. The resulting polyps, as they are called, can become so large that they fill the sinus completely and bulge into the nose. The polyps can usually be removed fairly simply using a snare. However, unless the conditions which caused the polyps to grow are dealt with, then they are likely to return.

Treatment to restore the drainage into the lymph system will ensure that the membrane shrinks, reducing the likelihood of a recurrence. One of the common problems associated with polyps in the maxillary sinus is snoring.

Josh, aged 38, had tried all sorts of remedies to stop his snoring – without any luck. His wife eventually persuaded him to come to my surgery to see if there was anything that I could do. When I examined him, I saw a polyp on the entrance to his left maxillary sinus and referred him to a surgeon who snared out a number of polyps in the sinuses on both sides. Josh had several treatments to the enlarged lymph nodes in his neck and was soon sleeping far more peacefully. When I saw him five years later, the polyps had not returned.

SKIN MAINTENANCE

Fluid retention and congestion caused by poor lymphatic drainage, particularly in the face or legs, can be unsightly and, over a prolonged period, leads tissues to age more rapidly. When the lymph nodes in the head and neck – which drain the face – are congested, the slight waterlogging of the tissues makes the complexion dull and can create shadows or bags under the eyes. Lymphatic drainage massage (see page 211) will help to clear blockages and tighten the skin as well as brightening up the complexion and making the skin appear more translucent (*see also* Cellulite).

Skin disorders can often be traced back to some dietary problem or food sensitivity, or to streptococcal infections in the throat spreading to and undermining the connective tissue of the skin.

SNORING

see Nightmares

SORE THROAT

see Laryngitis

SQUINTS

see Eye Conditions

STEROIDS

These are any substances that have cholesterol as their basic con-stituent. Steroids include many substances naturally produced by the body, as well as the corticosteroid and androsteroid drugs used by the medical profession to treat impotence in men and by athletes to build up muscles and enhance performance.

The risks associated with these drugs – including hormones like oestrogen and testosterone, which are all steroids – are often exagger-ated. There is nothing to fear in the steroids themselves, only in their misuse. Cortisone is probably one of the most valuable substances in the pharmacopoeia, capable of saving sight and preventing organs from becoming damaged when the body is in the throes of a disease. However, it is also used to mask symptoms of a disease which can cause considerable damage, as in the case of relieving the inflamma-tion that accompanies back pain. In the treatment of asthma, this treatment may suppress the body's own production of cortisone so that it is incapable of saving itself in an emergency.

In the old days – however bad an asthmatic spasm might be, even if the patient went blue – at the last moment before a fatal outcome the body would be flooded with cortisol, the bronchi would dilate and the life would be saved.

STICKY EYE

see Eye Conditions

STREPTOCOCCAL INFECTIONS

The word *streptococcus* simply means a chain of spherical 'bugs'. These are one of the most common of the bacterial invaders and some of the nastiest, particularly the haemolytic streptococci that cause 'strep' throat, tonsillitis and middle ear infection.

To penetrate the numerous defence mechanisms in the mouth and throat area, bacteria usually need to resort to extra weapons. The streptococcal variety have a number of toxins at their disposal for this purpose, designed to weaken the defences in the throat and ease the passage of the bacteria into the body.

STYE

see Eye Conditions – Conjunctivitis

SWOLLEN ANKLES AND KNEES

If you strain or twist your ankle or knee, then nature responds with an increased blood supply to initiate repair. However, if the neighbouring lymphatic nodes are blocked, this extra fluid has nowhere to drain, so the ankle or knee, after being swollen for a short period, do not settle and remain swollen. The resulting waterlogging further diminishes the repair mechanism and slows down the healing process.

Even when the fluid has drained, the ankle or knee can be vulnerable to a jolt or running or jumping action that would previously have had no effect. Ankles and knees are particularly prone to strains or twists, and, due to the increased blood supply, each additional injury further exacerbates the situation. The whole knee or ankle is weakened and swelling and pain may occur for no apparent reason.

It is not unusual for a person to experience the problem first in their mid-teens and, by the age of 20, be forced to give up all the activities that seem to bring the condition on. Often the ankle or knee remains trouble-free for some time, but the pain or swelling may suddenly reappear unexpectedly around the age of 40, following some mild exertion.

The recommended treatment is, first, rest, then a bandage or stocking, and exercises. Eventually, the fluid may be drained with a needle. In some instances surgical treatment may be required. For the majority of people these treatments are rarely satisfactory and they are saddled with permanently weakened ankles or knees.

In my experience, the problem is nearly always due to blocked lymph nodes in the groin. If these are treated, the problems usually clear up extremely rapidly. It is amazing how quickly repair can take place, even with quite marked degeneration in the knee resulting from softened and inadequately fed cartilages.

Phil was a very keen athlete. Around the age of 18, while playing football, he had twisted his knee very slightly when he was kicking the ball. It had became swollen and painful, but settled down after a week or so and he was able to carry on playing. He had no further problems until, nine months later, he was doing some exercises in the gym after a run and suddenly, for no apparent reason, his knee became swollen and painful again.

Once more, this settled with some anti-inflammatory drugs. However, only a few weeks later his knee swelled up again very early on in the course of game, and he was forced to abandon the match several times. His knee had been x-rayed and thoroughly examined at the hospital and he was told that it looked normal. There appeared to be no good explanation for the recurring problem.

When Phil came to me, I asked if he ever had athlete's foot, a question that I often ask people with knee troubles. It transpired that he had had a very bad case of athlete's foot, which was still not entirely cured after treatment. When I examined him, his knee was very slightly swollen, but he had full movement and the joint was stable.

There was no problem that could I could identify in the knee itself. However, when I looked at his groin I discovered that he had huge lymph nodes as a result of the constant debris being deposited from the infection in his toes. This had effectively blocked them, preventing the increased blood supply that followed the sprain to his knee from draining in the normal way, and so it accumulated around the knee in the form of swelling. This was the source of his complaint.

Phil had 11 treatments to the inguinal nodes over a period of several weeks. The lymph nodes never went right down, but they began to function much more effectively, and his knee became much more stable. He has returned from time to time in the four years since I first saw him with slight trouble. His lymph nodes remain slightly enlarged despite the treatment, so it is possible that he will always have a slight weakness in this knee, but it does not prevent him from playing lots of games and sport.

SYMPATHETIC NERVES

The automatic functions of the body are controlled by two separate nerve systems: the sympathetic and the parasympathetic. These are involved in a permanent 'tug-of-war' so if one stops working the other is left unopposed and becomes seriously overactive.

Back injuries in the thoracic area often cause a waterlogging of the sympathetic nerve 'computers', or ganglia, as they are called. This results in a low sympathetic drive which produces a number of symptoms, including tiredness and indigestion, and can be a significant factor in food sensitivities and absorptive problems. It should be considered as a possible component when these problems are being investigated. Treatment to the back will be needed if this diagnosis is made, otherwise the patient will never become completely well.

TEMPOROMANDIBULAR JOINT SYNDROME (TMJ)

TMJ, also known as temporomandibulitis, affects the temporo-mandibular joint which connects the substantial lower jaw bone to the comparatively small temporal bone of the skull, which means that it is fairly small and static on the one hand while, on the other, the huge chewing muscles exert enormous pressures on it. If the repair mechanism is not in good order, the following factors can increase the strain on this joint:

- Teeth that are irregular in length or do not meet each other correctly put a torsion strain on the joint which causes extra wear while eating.
- The tension in the shoulder and jaw muscles which often accompanies anxiety states places the joint under continuous stress.
- Wear and tear on the joint is intensified as sufferers often grind their teeth during the night.

The TMJ has several nerves that pass near it and which can become inflamed. This means that the symptoms can be distant from the joint and thus the cause not be suspected. So the syndrome is sometimes mistaken for ear trouble since it causes earache as well as facial aches, tenderness around the jaw (patients sometimes misguidedly end up having teeth removed because of the ache in the jaw) and pain lower down in the neck. It also commonly causes pain over the temple on that side. It is a condition which can cause a great deal of discomfort to patients such as 34-year-old Penny, who came to see me because she had a persistent toothache and a pain above her temple on the left side.

Penny said the pain was severe at times and especially bad at night. She was obviously in a rather tense state and had a lot of worries. She was not feeling very well in herself either. Penny had recently had two teeth out for the bad toothache, but unfortunately the pain persisted. At the time she also had pain down her neck, radiating around her throat. This often came at the same time as the pain over her temple. She had seen an ear, nose and throat specialist who told her there was nothing he could do.

I examined Penny and found that, when she opened her mouth, her jaw went slightly sideways as the jaw joint on the left side was rather stiff. I then put my finger onto the joint and pressed a little and she let out a yelp of pain. This made the diagnosis of temporomandibulitis quite certain.

Big nerves run right across the temporomandibular joint and, when the joint is inflamed, it is quite common to have referred pain in the teeth about half-way around the lower jaw. This is why her pain had not been relieved by removing those two teeth. The source of the ache was not in the teeth but in the jaw joint itself.

On examining her neck, I discovered that Penny had a number of enlarged lymph nodes, especially on the left side, that went down in a chain almost as far as her collarbone. She had treatment to these lymph nodes with ultrasonic waves and an electrical current to make the muscles in her face on that side contract and force fluid through the lymph nodes.

Penny's jaw joint was gently stretched to improve the movement and help relieve some of the pain. She was also given an anti-inflammatory pill to ease the inflammation of the joint. After the first few treatments the joint became much less tender. She was given 11 treatments in all and made a very good recovery. All the pains subsided and she felt much better in herself and generally clearer in her head.

The conventional treatment for temporomandibulitis is to put in a dental plate to even up the balance of the pressures on the teeth; another is to give tranquillizing pills to reduce the effects of the stress. The best method, in my opinion, is to restore the lymph drainage to the area; this is often all that is needed to cure the condition. Electrical treatment over the actual joint itself is often helpful. This problem in the joint is also commonly associated with trouble in the stellate ganglion at the base of the neck, associated with an old neck injury. This can upset the function of this nerve system. If so, this needs to be corrected.

TINNITUS

see Ear Problems

TOXINS

These are chemicals produced by bacteria and released into the body. They result in swelling or damage – even of the membranes of the throat or skin. Toxins can also be poisons that are absorbed through the skin or membrane. The toxins produced by bacteria are either *endo toxins*, which are inside the bacterium and become a problem if the bacteria disintegrate, or *exo toxins*, which are secreted by the bacteria as an aid to their own survival. The streptococcal bacteria are capable of putting out a toxin that inflames the membranes similar to those in the mouth (that is, to the membranes lining joints), and sometimes muscles, connective tissue and skin.

TRAVEL SICKNESS

This is generally due to trouble in the inner ear, which affects balance and the detection of movement. Because of the connection between the ear and the vagus nerve – responsible for over-activity in the stomach – the conflict resolves itself by the patient feeling sick and sometimes vomiting. A person is more likely to suffer from travel sickness if the ear is slightly congested. Lymph drainage treatment to the lymph nodes in the neck will often alleviate this problem.

ULCERS

Ulcers are due to a breakdown of the surface tissue, either in the skin or the mucous membranes. Stomach and duodenal ulcers (also known as peptic ulcers) are a special case as they are often brought about by a malfunction of the autonomic nervous system. The faulty working of the sympathetic nervous system allows the parasympathetic to overwork, pouring acid continuously into the stomach, so that it burns a hole in itself. It also increases the contractions that churn the food up and push digested food into the duodenum. If this happens too fast through over-activity, it may burn a hole in the wall of the duodenum, causing a duodenal ulcer. The heliobacter bacteria are resistant to acid and can infect an ulcer. This may require antibiotic treatment.

Lymphatic drainage treatment to the area around the 'nerve computer' in the middle of the chest area will often clear up these ulcers permanently (*see* Irritable Bowel Syndrome).

Leg ulcers are caused by a number of factors, including poor circulation, diabetes and varicose veins. The weight of the column of blood from the heart to the ankles is fairly considerable, and the task of getting the blood and lymph back to the heart from these areas poses a physical problem. There is a huge plexus of veins in the middle of the sole of the foot which is squeezed at every step, resulting in a huge pumping of blood back up the veins. The contraction of the calf and thigh muscles also creates a powerful pumping action. Under ordinary conditions, this mechanism is more than adequate to ensure a good circulation.

However, the valves in the superficial veins are fragile and not well supported by surrounding tissues, and if subjected to excessive pressure will bulge and leak blood into the segment beneath, where it pools, doubling the pressure on the valve below and causing it, too, to become incompetent. This means there is now three times the pressure on the next valve down, and so the condition of varicose veins spreads. It is for this reason that I believe that the problem should be treated as early as possible. The devitalization of the tissues resulting from the reduction in supplies of oxygen and other nutrients carried by the blood can lead to the formation of ulcers, and can also make them difficult to treat and slow to heal.

Lymphatic drainage treatment targeted above the affected area, concentrating particularly on enlarged and congested lymph nodes in the groin, usually brings about a rapid improvement in the tissues and the healing of the ulcer. Problems in the veins also need addressing – usually by surgery.

Desmond, aged 43, had come to me about his bad back. In the course of treatment he told me that he was very bothered by some ulcers and eczema on the calf of his right leg, which were both unsightly and irritable. When the eczema broke down into ulcers, of which there were about eight, these were very sore.

He had had treatment over a period of six years in all for this, but the condition had very slowly deteriorated. I examined his leg and found that he had very enlarged lymph nodes in his groin. I suggested lymphatic drainage treatment to reduce these, as well as ultrasound to the ulcers themselves. The swelling in the lymph nodes did go down, although not to a completely normal level. The eczema also receded to about one-fifth of its original area and was no longer affected by ulcers, but it refused to improve any further than that.

ULTRASONIC WAVES

see Dolphins

VARICOSE VEINS

see Ulcers

VESTIBULITIS

see Ear Problems

VITAMINS

These are substances which have been found to be essential for the healthy functioning of the body. Serious deficiencies are closely associated with certain diseases. Vitamins A and D can cause problems if they are taken to excess, whereas other vitamins tend to be excreted if optimum levels are exceeded. (See chapter 4 for further details.)

PART
IV

LYMPHATIC DRAINAGE TREATMENTS

When your lymphatic system is treated using the techniques described below, the blockages which cause the body to break down in the first place – and subsequently delay the process of recovery – are cleared. Many people are surprised at the wide range of diseases that can be treated simply by restoring defective lymphatic drainage in the affected area. So many patients say that they have tried all sorts of treatments for their specific ailment, with little joy. Sometimes they have been told that they must simply learn to live with their condition. To me, this is often unacceptable. Provided it has not become too advanced, there may well be something that can be done to help.

The parts of the lymphatic mechanism most often affected are the groups of lymph nodes that drain large areas and often varied parts of the body. The problem is almost always the same – these lymph nodes have been overloaded by the products of disease and, in their capacity as filters, they have become partially blocked. This leads, as we have seen, both to problems from the back-pressure of fluid overwhelming the drainage area as a whole and to a weakened response of the lymph nodes to the presence of infection. This therefore may well involve structures not involved in the original problem.

Unless they are very swollen, lymph nodes can be hard to detect until you acquire the knack. Some people describe the texture beneath the skin as feeling like semolina, others like broad beans. The rule of thumb is that, if you are aware of even the slightest swelling in a spot where you would expect to find a lymph node, then it is substantially enlarged.

The cervical nodes are often more prominent if the patient is lying down. Congested inguinal nodes are easier to spot than most.

Treatment varies according to the complaint and the accessibility of the area concerned, but any – or a combination – of the following may be needed:

- the forms of physical medicine outlined below to improve local conditions and assist the body's defence and repair mechanism

- dietary supplements and drugs to restore deficiencies – often brought about by the illness itself. These might include vitamins, minerals and trace elements, such as iron or zinc, and even hormones.

- addressing associated or underlying problems, such as food sensitivities

- advice on external factors that may be contributing to the problem, such as overclothing and overheating in the case of asthma and other respiratory problems, or an unsuitable diet in the case of someone with gastric problems

- measures to improve the overall health of the patient, such as targeted exercises

- special measures for specific diseases, such as cold baths to reactivate the sympathetic nervous system in the case of ME sufferers, have met with only doubtful success

- drugs designed actively to assist the elimination of the disease, such as anti-inflammatory drugs for arthritis, or an antibiotic if the primary problem is an infection

■ removal of irreparably damaged parts of the lymphatic system. The most obvious examples are infected tonsils and adenoids, or a damaged appendix. Much less common would be the removal of badly damaged lymph nodes – or a single node.

TREATMENT

Treatment to the lymph nodes can take various forms. Massage, ultrasound and electrical muscle stimulation are the methods I will discuss here.

MASSAGE

Massage is a simple and effective way of decongesting the lymph nodes and improving the flow of lymphatic fluid through them. It is also a technique that can easily be carried out at home with impressive results.

Lymphatic drainage massage involves moderately firm pressure and a sort of vibrating rotating action, often using just the first two or three fingers. Although the experience may be more pleasurable with lubrication, the friction generated by direct skin-to-skin contact has a greater impact on underlying tissues. You should always follow the natural direction of drainage – that is, towards the heart.

Ideally, massage for five minutes once or twice daily until the lymph nodes return to their normal size – a timer can be useful here. The sensation should not be painful, although there may be slight discomfort if the lymph nodes are tender. You can successfully treat lymphatic blockages in the head, neck and groin yourself. Massaging the thoracic nodes at the root of the lung is also very worthwhile, especially if there is an asthmatic in the family, although it is harder to carry this out on yourself.

You should notice some improvement after two or three sessions, although you will need to carry on the treatment for a minimum of three weeks to achieve lasting results. Think in terms of three months or so for asthmatic conditions.

ULTRASOUND

Ultrasound treatment cannot be done at home, but needs to be carried out by a qualified doctor, physiotherapist, osteopath or chiropractor.

High-frequency sound waves are used to break up the debris lodged within the lymph nodes, so that it can be removed piecemeal or dissolved at a later stage. Ultrasonic treatment covers the same area as the massage. Ultrasound is also thought to reduce inflammation and speed up the healing process. The deeper penetration of longwave ultrasound is particularly useful for treating conditions affecting the lungs, such as asthma, bronchitis and emphysema, and the deep-seated abdominal nodes.

ELECTRICAL MUSCLE STIMULATION

Electrical treatment cannot be done at home, but needs to be carried out by a qualified doctor, physiotherapist, osteopath or chiropractor.

Also known as surged faradism, electrical muscle stimulation involves a rhythmical pumping action achieved by passing an electric current between two electrodes applied at different points on the skin over the nerves that supply the muscles surrounding the congested lymph node. This works on the same principle as a rubber plunger clearing the drain of a kitchen sink, driving the backed-up water in the sink in explosive bursts down the pipe to break up the mass, and then propelling it down into the waste pipe.

The effect on the immediate area is to drive the fluid lying in the tissue spaces, in one co-ordinated pulse, down the ducts that lead to the affected nodes. This is achieved by setting up a repeating cycle of contraction and relaxation in the surrounding muscles.

This treatment should be carried out for two or three minutes at a time.

Now let's look at some guidelines for treating ailments associated with blockages of the main groups of lymph nodes, using all of the techniques described above.

HEAD AND NECK

GENERAL CONGESTION/SINUSES/HAY FEVER/EAR PROBLEMS

Massage

Start between the eyebrows, rubbing very gently across the top of each eyebrow (see Fig 1) and round the eyes until you reach the edge of the nose.

Next, massage from the outer corner of the nostrils over the lower part of the cheekbones (see Fig 2), down towards the angle of the jaw.

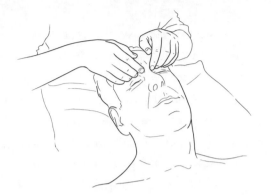

FIG 1

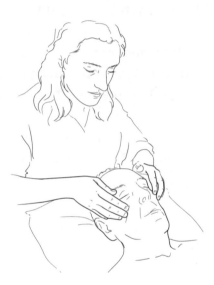

FIG 2

Then, using a small zig-zag movement and increasing the pressure, work your way down the chain of lymph nodes that starts just behind the angle of the jaw and finishes at the collarbone. These are the cervical groups of nodes.

Continue for about five minutes.

The aim is to push the lymph down through these nodes and back to the big vessels at the root of the neck.

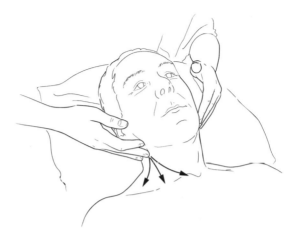

FIG 3

For ear problems, work the area in front of the ear, just below the outer edge of the cheekbone and behind the ear, about halfway up.

Drain down towards the angle of the jaw (see Fig 3) where the tonsil nodes lie. (When the tonsil nodes are involved in illness, they will be felt as firm lozenge shapes roughly two times their normal size.) Then massage in a diagonal down towards the collarbone.

Ultrasound

Normal ultrasonic waves are useful for treating both groups of lymph nodes in the neck, starting at the mastoid process and moving down to the nodes just above the clavicle. Each side should be treated for about three minutes.

The new longer-wave ultrasound penetrates into the sinuses and inner ear. Applying it over the maxillary and frontal sinuses and around the ear can be beneficial.

Electrical Treatment

This can be very effective in treating ailments in this area. Apply the pads in the following way:

1 One on either side of base of the neck, right across the seventh cervical vertebra, to boost the circulation around the stellate ganglion. This controls the blood supply to the sinuses. Treat for three minutes.

2 Leave one on the neck and place another on the facial nerve, about 1–2 inches in front of the earlobe, just over the temporo-mandibular joint. The current should produce a significant contraction of the facial muscles and a milder one in the muscles of the neck. Treat both sides together for three minutes.

3 One on the neck and another just above the dip where the forehead and nose meet – over the ciliary ganglion. When the current is applied the patient will feel a great deal of pressure under the pad in the nose, and it usually comes on suddenly. It is therefore important that the machine should be set slowly so that the sensation is comfortable. One minute is sufficient in this area.

EYES

GLAUCOMA/RETINAL DETACHMENT/ CATARACTS/ CONJUNCTIVITIS

Massage

Massage very gently from the inner corner of the eye, over the upper and lower lids and down over the cheekbones (see Fig 4) towards the tonsil nodes.

Then drain downwards through the lymph glands in the neck (see diagram). With infectious conditions like conjunctivitis, it is important to wash your hands very thoroughly after contact.

Ultrasound

Use weaker strength (1–3 MHz) and treat for 1–2 minutes as per massage.

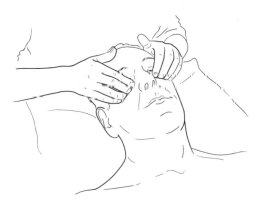

FIG 4

Electrical Treatment

Place one pad on the neck and the other just below the outer corner of the eye. The current, which must remain at a comfortable level – increase very slowly – should produce a movement of the whole of the extrinsic muscles of the eye, which will be seen to 'twitch'. Treat each eye separately for three minutes.

The second pad should then be applied to the ciliary ganglion at the root of the nose for one minute.

THROAT AND LARYNX

(See diagram, page 63.)

Massage

Massage both groups of lymph nodes in the neck for five minutes, starting with the tonsil node, located behind the angle of the jaw, and moving down towards the nodes situated just above the collarbone.

When the tonsils are involved in disease, the tonsil nodes become very hard and enlarged and can be markedly tender.

For conditions involving the larynx, massage over the front of the neck and larynx, about 1 inch above the collarbone, towards the lymph nodes at the back of the triangles formed by the ear and the collarbone. Continue for about five minutes.

Ultrasound

Apply ultrasound to the cervical lymph nodes and the larynx, if this is part of the problem, for approximately five minutes.

Electrical Treatment

The electrical treatment for problems in the throat area involves applying two pads over the stellate ganglion, and leaving one there. Then two pads should be applied on either side of the neck, just below the angle of the jaw, for three minutes either side. This should stimulate a contraction of all the muscles of the neck.

TRACHEA (WINDPIPE)

LARYNGITIS/BRONCHITIS/EMPHYSEMA

This usually involves the lower group of lymph nodes in the neck and those in the hilar region of the lungs (see diagram on page 63).

Massage

Massage helps to decongest and reduce any muscle spasm in the area. Start either side of the trachea and drain downwards, working the triangles formed on either side of the neck – by the ears at the top and the collarbone at the base.

Ultrasound

Apply ultrasonic waves to the hilar region for five minutes. If longer-wave ultrasound is available, this should be given over the front of the lungs as it penetrates deeply enough to assist the bronchi by breaking up the mucus. Five minutes is generally sufficient, although chronic cases may benefit from up to ten minutes.

In addition, the pads should be placed either side of the spine over the hilar region for three minutes.

THE LUNGS/ASTHMA

Lung problems and asthma almost invariably involve the upper respiratory tract as well, so follow treatment for sinus and throat trouble (see above) as well as for the lungs.

Massage

The thoracic spine should be massaged using a firm rotating motion for about five minutes (see Fig 5).

With asthma, some mobilization of the thoracic vertebrae and ribs is usually necessary as they have a tendency to seize up. Have the patient lie on her stomach and apply pressure – such as that generated by standing to one side and leaning your weight onto one hand pressed on top of the other and pushing down smartly across the back of the patient's ribcage, moving from the top to the bottom of the ribcage (see Fig 6). This helps to expand the ribs on the front of the body as well.

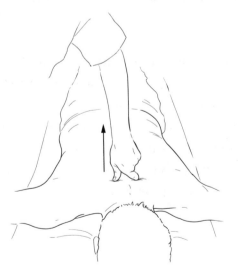

FIG 5

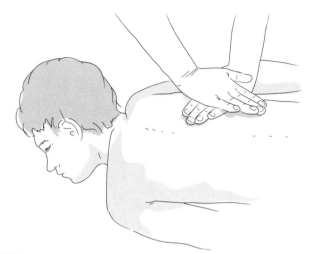

FIG 6

Ultrasound

Apply ultrasonic waves over the hilar area for five minutes. If longer-wave ultrasound is available, it is useful to treat the front of the chest for five to ten minutes as well, as this can help to relieve spasms in the bronchi.

Place pads on either side of the hilar region for three minutes.

In cases of emphysema, treatment need be given to the lung area only – that is, hilar pads and ultrasound over the front of the chest. Massage and mobilization of the thoracic spine is also beneficial (see diagram on page 220). Longwave ultrasound is also of great benefit, as for asthma.

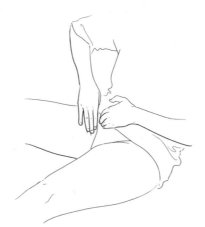

FIG 7

ABDOMEN

CYSTITIS/UTERINE PROBLEMS/RECURRENT VULVAL INFECTIONS

Massage

Massage the inguinal nodes (best performed lying on back) on the upper side of the inguinal ligament. If the nodes on the lower side of the ligament are large, these should be treated too, as they drain the lower part of the abdomen and the perineum. Massage to the small of the back (by another person) is also helpful. Continue for five minutes in each location.

Ultrasound

Apply ultrasonic waves to the inguinal nodes for about five minutes on each side, and to the mid-lumbar region of the spine to treat the congestion around the lumbar nodes. Longwave ultrasound up and down the middle of the abdomen for five minutes will also be extremely beneficial.

Electrical Treatment

Give electrical treatment through pads in the mid-lumbar region for three minutes.

LEGS

INFECTIONS/ATHLETE'S FOOT/ULCERS

Massage

Massage treatment is mainly to the lymph nodes on the lower side of the inguinal ligament for about five minutes, although it is advisable to massage the ones on the upper side as well (see Fig 8).

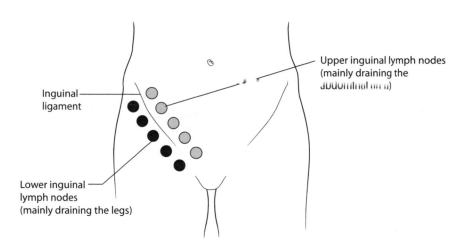

Inguinal ligament

Upper inguinal lymph nodes (mainly draining the abdominal area)

Lower inguinal lymph nodes (mainly draining the legs)

FIG 8

Ultrasound

Apply ultrasound over the inguinal nodes for five minutes. Ulcers may benefit from being treated with the longwave ultrasound instrument, if available, for the same length of time. This can be applied to the opposite side of the leg initially and then, when the wound begins to heal, it can be applied directly.

Electrical Treatment

Electrical treatment to the quadriceps definitely improves drainage from the leg. One long, sticky electrode is placed either side of the thigh.

Supplements

In cases where wounds are healing poorly, large doses of vitamin C – up to 2 grams a day – for several weeks can be of enormous help.

Local or systemic treatment to clear up the infection, whether it is bacterial or fungal, will help to speed up the effect of the treatment.

ARTHRITIC OR SPRAINED JOINTS

KNEE PROBLEMS

- massage the lymph nodes in the inguinal region for three minutes
- ultrasound to the knee-ankle and inguinal nodes for five minutes each
- electrical treatment to the quadriceps for three minutes
- mobilization and traction of the knee
- advising the patient to raise the leg for a period of time every day to improve drainage

■ an elastic bandage, where necessary, to encourage drainage up the veins and lymphatics

SPRAINED ANKLE

A common reason for a delayed recovery with a sprained ankle is that the synovial membrane becomes trapped in the joint. The membrane is a loose cover around the joint, which allows free movement in relation to the surrounding tissues. When the sprain separates the two surfaces of the joint, usually on the front, this membrane falls into the space and is trapped as the bones come together.

In this situation, physiotherapy mimicking the original sprain needs to be given to stretch the skin and tissues and release the synovial membrane, which gives instant relief. However, because the membrane becomes swollen and moulded to the shape of the joint, it can become trapped again and the treatment may well need to be repeated. A cold spray and treatment with ultrasound to stop it from swelling will help to avoid this.

ARMS

Problems with the arms are rare, but a wound can sometimes be slow to heal. In this case, the lymph nodes in the armpit require treatment with massage and ultrasound for five minutes. If the wound is in the hand area, electrical treatment to the muscles of the arm for three minutes greatly improves the drainage from the whole of the arm.

GLOSSARY

Abdomen The cavity of the body containing the large internal organs

Abdominal Relating to the abdomen

Acute An illness with intense symptoms and a short duration

Adenoids A mass of lymphoid tissue at the back of the nose and throat, above the tonsils

Adrenal glands Glands on top of the kidneys that secrete adrenaline and cortisol

Adrenaline Secretion of adrenal gland that mimics sympathetic activity

Allergy Heightened reaction to an antigen

Alveolus/i Air cells of the lung

Antibody Protein manufactured by lymphocytes to neutralize or destroy antigen

Antigen A substance in bacteria, viruses and other micro-organisms that stimulates the production of antibodies

Appendix A blind, narrow tube leading off the caecum

Arterial Referring to the arteries

Artery A vessel carrying blood from the heart

Arthritis Inflammation of a joint

Asthma Spasms of the bronchial tubes leading to breathing difficulties

Athlete's foot Fungal infection between the toes

Autonomic nervous system The sympathetic and parasympathetic nervous systems that control all systems not under conscious control

Bacteria Micro-organisms capable of independent existence

Bell's palsy Acute facial paralysis

Binocular vision The ability to join the slightly dissimilar images of the two eyes into one final image

Bladder Bag into which urine passes from the kidneys

Bronchi The two main air passages to each lung

Bronchiole Small air tube

Bronchitis Inflammation of the bronchial tree

Bruise Blood in the tissues from an injury

Caecum Blind tube off the large bowel

Candida Yeast infection causing thrush and other infections

Capillary Length of minute vessels joining the smallest arterioles to venules through which tissue fluid diffuses

Carbon dioxide Gas produced by metabolism and exchanged in the lungs for oxygen

Cataract Opacity of the lens of the eye

Catarrh Inflammation of a mucus membrane causing an increase in the amount of mucus secreted

Cellulose The principal constituent of plant cell walls

Chronic Disease lasting a long period of time

Cochlea The snail shell-like spiral of the inner ear containing the hearing mechanism

Conjunctiva The mucus membrane lining the eyelids

Cornea Transparent front part of the covering of the eyeball

Cortisol The hormone produced by the outer layer of the adrenal gland

Cortisone The synthetic version of cortisol; also the active breakdown product from cortisol

Cysterna chyli Large lymphatic duct which plays a part in the transport of fats

Cystitis Inflammation of the urinary bladder

Dermatitis An often non-infective disease of the skin of known causation – see Eczema

Devitalized (of tissue) All its functions diminished, most importantly its ability to resist invaders

Diabetes A disease of excessive blood sugar caused by inadequate supplies of insulin

Diffuse To extend or spread widely

Diverticulitis Inflammation of the diverticula in the colon

Diverticulosis The presence of diverticula in the colon

Diverticula Small sacs or pouches in the inner wall of the colon

Eczema A usually non-contagious inflammatory disease of the skin of unknown origin

Electroencephalogram The making of a graphic record of the electrical impulses of the brain

Emphysema A condition where the alveoli of the lungs are dilated and almost useless

Epilepsy Fits caused by malfunction of the brain

Eustachian tube A pressure-equalizing tube going from the throat to the middle ear

Fallopian tubes The tubes that collect the ovum from the ovary and pass it to the uterus

Faradism surged An interrupted electrical current with a rhythmical change of intensity

Ganglia Minute multi-tasking computers found all over the body which control blood pressure, blood sugar, repair, maintenance, secretions, etc. Also swelling on a tendon sheath

Glaucoma A condition caused by increased pressure within the eye

Haemoglobin The pigment in red blood cells that transports oxygen

Hereditary Transmitted from ancestors or parents to child by DNA

HypoSympathetic Tone (HST) A condition that is caused by underactivity of the sympathetic nervous system; often caused by back trouble

Inguinal Relating or belonging to the groin, or in the region of the groin

Inner ear A series of membranous sacs and ducts which are responsible for the perception sound and balance

Ions Atoms bearing an electrical charge

Laryngitis Inflammation of the larynx

Larynx The organ in the throat responsible for voice production

Laxative A remedy to loosen faeces or to increase the peristalsis in the bowel

Leucocyte/s *see White cells, below*

Leukaemia A sometimes fatal disease of the white blood cells

Lomotil A drug to stop diarrhoea

Longwave ultrasound Lower frequency ultra-sonic waves

Lymph A pale, yellow, clear (or cloudy) fluid flowing in lymphatic channels

Lymphatic Relating to, secreting or conveying lymph

Lymph nodes Popularly referred to as 'glands', these are the combined filtering stations and chemical factories that produce antibodies designed to destroy bacteria, viruses and foreign bodies and neutralize toxins. There are various conglomerations of lymph nodes strategically located around the body. When lymph nodes become obstructed, it causes congestion in the tissues, which affects their ability to resist and overcome infection

Lymphocytes Type of white blood cell incorporated into tailor-made immune response against organisms which penetrate the body's general defences

Massage Manual manipulation of the bodily tissues

Mastoid Air channels in the skull beneath and connected to the ear. Part of the sinus complex

Membrane A thin layer of tissue which covers or divides a space or organ

Menière's disease Dizzy attacks, deafness and noises in the ear

Metabolism Chemical processes essential for life

Middle ear Between the outer and inner drums of the ear; contains the three ossicles (bones that magnify sound). Joined to the throat by the Eustachian tube

Mucous glands Glands in the mucous membranes which secrete mucus

Mucus The viscous secretion of mucous membrane

Muscle pump The squeezing effect of a contracting muscle to return blood from the periphery of the body to the heart

Node A swelling – usually a lymph node that can be felt

Ophthalmic Relating to the eye

Ossicles Three joining bones of the ear which transmit and magnify sound across the middle ear

Oxygen A colourless, odourless and tasteless gas in the atmosphere. Necessary for life

Peristalsis A propelling wave of contraction in a muscular tube

Peritonitis Inflammation of the peritoneal membrane

Physiotherapy Treatment by physical means – massage, manipulation, electrical and sound waves

Pink-eye Inflammation of the conjunctiva of the eye

Polyps Extensions arising from swollen mucous membranes

Psychological Associated with the mind

Red cells Red blood cells that carry oxygen to the tissues and carbon dioxide from them back to the lungs

Retina Light-sensitive lining of the back of the eye

Salpingitis Inflammation of the ovary tubes

Scurvy A disease caused by lack of vitamin C. Today bleeding gums is often a very mild version

Semicircular canals Balance mechanism of the inner ear. They register movement of the head in all directions

Serotonin A chemical messenger found in the body and brain

Sinus Cavities in the skull including the antrum and ear

Splanchnic ganglion One of the sympathetic nerve centres, largely supplying the stomach

Spore Seed of a fungus

Stellate ganglion One of the 'little brains' of the sympathetic nerve system. Lies on the muscles at the base of the neck

Stereoscope Optical apparatus to detect presence of stereoscopic vision. Also used to train people lacking stereoscopic vision and to visualize stereoscopic pictures

Steroid Chemicals made of cholesterol including sex hormones, bile acid, cortisone and vitamin D

Streptococcus Round bacterium joined together like beads

Surged Faradism See Faradism

Sympathetic nervous system With the parasympathetic, makes up the autonomic system that controls and works all the automatic functions of the body

Tinea pedis Fungus causing athlete's foot

Tinnitus Noises in the ear

Tissue fluid Fluid bathing tissue cells

Tonsil Lymph complex in the throat. Forming a first line of defence against bacterial and virus attacks – not needed after the age of seven or so

Toxin Any biological poison

Trachea Windpipe

Tympanic membrane Eardrum

Ulcer Break in the surface of a membrane

Ultrasonic waves A very high frequency sound wave, usually from 700,000 to 3,000,000 a second

Uterus Womb

Varicose ulcer Ulcer in the leg caused by a varicose vein and poor circulation brought about by the blood flowing the wrong way down varicose veins

Varicose vein A vein with incompetent valves circulating the blood in the wrong direction

Vestibule A cavity in the inner ear with stones in it to enable a sense of the precise positioning of the head

Virus A microscopic organism – so small that it has to depend on its host for nutrition, unlike a bacterium which is independent

Vulva The female external genitalia

White cells White cells found in the blood, tissue space and lymphatic system. Also known as leucocytes

INDEX

A-Z directory of problems 119-206
abdomen 221-2
abdominal adenitis 77
abdominal nodes 93, 95-7, 137
acidophilus 51
additives 43
adenoids 4, 5, 18, 19-21, 61, 72-3, 211
adrenal glands 52, 111, 172
air conditioning 40-1, 101, 113
air pressure imbalances 87
allergic asthma 103, 123-4
allergies 26, 51, 53, 65, 152, 171-2, 174
alternatives 53
alveoli 99-100, 102, 154-5
ankles 26, 198-200, 225
anti-bacterial products 43
anti-inflammatories 28, 51, 199, 202,
    210
antibiotics 3-4, 17, 26, 39
  abuse 46-51
  debate 46-51
  guidelines 50-1
  lymphatic time line 45
  tonsils 64
antibodies 13, 15, 16-17, 19-20
  breastfeeding 43
  children 44
  food 42-3
  lymphatic system 22
  overload 102

repair 26
swollen membranes 25, 27
thoracic nodes 100
antigens 15
appendicitis 75, 121-2, 176
appendix 5, 9, 13, 18
  lymphatic structure 20-2, 61, 67,
    73-81
  treatment 211
appetite 122-3
aqua-aerobics 32
arms 225
arthritis 6, 142-4, 187-9, 224-5
asthma 6, 8, 36, 65, 98
  lymphatic malfunction 123-6
  overload 102-18
  steroids 197
  treatment 210, 220-1
athlete's foot 12, 24, 94, 97
  lymphatic malfunction 126-7,
    199-200
  treatment 223-4

babies 20, 30-1, 34-7, 43
  asthma 112
  body temperature 130
  cot death 134-5
  lymphatic time line 46
  thoracic nodes 100
back pain 33, 79-80, 184-5, 197

bacteria 5, 9, 10, 12
    antibiotics 49
    defence mechanisms 19
    sterilization 43
    sugar 55
    swollen membranes 25-6
    tonsils 61, 63
    useful 16, 51
bedclothes 35
Bells' facial palsy 127-9
bladder 23, 76, 95-7, 136-7
blepharitis 158-9
blocked tear ducts 159-60
blood circulation 11-12
body temperature 33-7, 130
boils 13
bowel 18, 22, 51, 61, 67
    abdominal nodes 97
    appendix 73, 75, 77, 79, 80-1
    irritable bowel syndrome 175-7
    wheat 172
brain 67-8, 108, 187
breastfeeding 20, 43, 53, 130
breathing 32, 83, 98, 111
    emphysema 154-6
    overload 114-17
bronchitic asthma 103-7, 110-11
    lymphatic malfunction
        124-6
    overload 113-14
bronchitis 6, 8, 45, 65, 98
    asthma 112, 118
    lymphatic malfunction 124-6, 131

caecum 21-2
canals 86-7
candida 51
case studies 17, 21, 36
    adenoids 72-3
    antibiotics 47-8, 50

appendix 78-9, 79-80
arthritis of ossicles 143-4
asthma 103, 106-7, 108-9, 112-14
athlete's foot 127
Bells' facial palsy 128-9
blepharitis 159
cataracts 161
congestion 65-6
conjunctivitis 162-3
cystitis 136-7
deafness 146-7
detached retina 165
dizziness 145-6
ears 88
eczema 153-4
epilepsy 157-8
glaucoma 166
inguinal nodes 94-5
lymphatic time line 45
Ménière's disease 150-1
mental function 68-9
middle ear 141
painful periods 184-5
positive ions 39-40
rheumatoid arthritis 188-9
salpingitis 189-90
short sight 168-9
sinusitis 193-4, 195
squints 170-1
swollen knees 199-200
temporomandibular joint syndrome
    202
tinnitus 148-9
ulcers 205-6
cataracts 160-1, 217-18
catarrh 39-40, 51, 65-7, 88, 102, 131
cellulite 131-2
cellulose 21
central heating 40, 101, 112, 210
cerebral oedema 132-3, 187

cervical nodes 82-91, 118, 163, 210
children 20, 33, 34-7, 40-1
  antibiotics 48
  appendix 76-8
  asthma 104-9, 112
  body temperature 130
  clothing 101, 152
  diet 53-4
  immune system 42
  lymphatic time line 44-6, 46
  mental function 67
  supplements 56-7
  thoracic nodes 100
  tonsils 64-5
cigarettes 101-2
circulation 11-12
clothing 34-7, 65, 101, 112-13, 130,
    134-5, 210
cochlea 86
coffee 172, 175
colds 4, 39-40, 45, 47, 69
  ear problems 88
  tonsils 70
colostrum 20
congestion 65-7, 102, 110-11, 213-16
conjunctiva 90
conjunctivitis 162-3, 217-18
constipation 80-1, 133
cooling mechanisms 33-7
cortisol 51, 111, 172
cortisone 52, 110-11, 174, 197
cot death 130, 134-5
cow's milk 3, 53, 114, 130
  eczema 152, 154
  lymphatic malfunction 134-5, 172,
    175
cysterna chyli 97
cystitis 3, 6, 76, 135-7, 221-2

dairy 52-3

damaged tonsils 62-3, 67, 69-75
  cervical nodes 84
  eczema 152
  nightmares 183
  treatment 211
deafness 145-7
defence mechanisms 13, 18, 42, 45, 61
dental problems 138
detached retina 164-5, 217-18
diabetes 163
diesel 101
diet 51-8, 79-81, 111, 114, 135, 210
digestive system 22, 52-3, 56
directory of problems 119-206
diverticulosis 80
dizziness 145-7
dolphins 139
dowager's hump 139-40
drink 12, 18, 42

ears 6, 13, 17, 21, 27
  antibiotics 48, 50
  cervical nodes 83
  lifestyle 33, 47
  problems 84-8, 140-51, 213-16
  repair 27
eczema 3, 6, 85, 135, 151-4
electrical muscle stimulation 9, 28, 65
  asthma 118
  treatments 212-13, 216, 218-19, 222,
    224-5
elimination diet 52
emphysema 154-6
epilepsy 156-8
Eustachian tube 86-8
evolution 10
exercise 31-3, 112, 210
eyes 6, 89-91, 158-71, 217-18

face 26

faeces 44
fibrous tissue 13
food 12, 18, 42-3
    abdominal nodes 96
    appendix 79-80
    intolerances 67
food manufacturers 43
food poisoning 43
food sensitivity 17-7, 51-2, 69, 80
    lymphatic malfunction 140, 152,
        171-2
    overload 102
    treatment 210
foreign bodies 12-13
fresh air 33-4, 40, 65, 101, 112, 152
fungi 12, 43, 51, 55
fur 33, 34, 36, 130

gastritis 67, 80
glands 16
glandular fever 172
glaucoma 165-7, 217-18
glue ear 142
gluten 172, 175
groin 17, 94, 95, 137, 199-200
guide to lymphatic system 10-22
gums 96, 138

hands 26
hay fever 26, 66, 88, 173-4, 213-16
head 213-16
heating see central heating
hormone replacement therapy 139-40
hygiene 42, 44

immune system 13, 42
infections 5, 7-8, 11, 16-17
    antibiotics 46-51
    babies 30-1
    blockages 23-4

defence mechanisms 20-2, 42
    streptococcal 151, 198
    tonsils 61-2
infective bronchitic asthma 103-7,
    110-11, 124-6
influenza 45, 107
inguinal nodes 93-5, 97, 200
inner ear 86-7, 144-51
intestines 16
ionization 175
irritable bowel syndrome 175-7

joint pain 177-8
joints 224-5

kidneys 96, 136
knees 198-200, 224-5

laryngitis 6, 178-9
larynx 218-19
laxatives 97
leg ulcers 94, 204-6, 223-4
lifestyle 30-1, 44, 101-18
lines of defence 3-9
lungs 24, 33, 36, 39
    cervical nodes 83
    overload 102
    thoracic nodes 99
    treatment 220-1
lymph nodes 5, 7-9, 14-19, 22-4
lymphatic system 4-8, 10-22
    breakdown 23-9
    directory of problems
        119-206
    drainage 8-9
    overload 16, 101-18
    repair 23-9
    treatment 207-25
lymphatic time line 46
lymphocytes 11, 15, 22, 102

magnesium 181-2
malfunction directory 119-206
management of asthma 111-18
massage 9, 28, 65, 118, 211-15, 217-25
membranes 180-1
Menière's disease 150-1
menstruation 184-5
mental function 67-8
middle ear 86, 140-2
minerals 57-8, 181-2, 210
Moon 40
movement 31-3
mucus 12, 13, 65, 74
multiple sclerosis 182
muscle guarding 77

nausea 182-3
neck 213-16
nightmares 183
nose 13, 33, 36, 39-40

ophthalmic surgeons 164
ossicles 142-4
osteomyelitis 183-4
osteoporosis 139
outer ear 85
overheating 34-7
overload 101-18
painful periods 184-5
panting 33, 35
pavement cells 24
periods 184-5
peritoneum 22, 75
peritonitis 75, 185-6
Peyer's patches 18, 97
physical medicine 111, 118, 210
physiotherapists 9, 27, 95, 164
Pilates 32
pink-eye 162
poisons 12

pollens 101, 173-4
pollution 38-41, 101, 174
polyps 186
positive ions 38-41, 175
prostaglandin 28-9
psychological problems 108-9, 187

recommended daily amount (RDA) 56,
    182
removal of tonsils 69-72, 211
respiratory system 98-100
retina 164-5, 217-18
rheumatoid arthritis 187-9

salpingitis 189-90
scarlet fever 190
scurvy 57, 138
sedentary lifestyles 31-3
self-help 30-58
sell-by dates 43
septicaemia 17
serotonin 39, 175
shingles 191
short sight 167-9
sick building syndrome 41
sinuses 6, 8, 13, 25, 39-40
    cervical nodes 83
    self-help 45, 51
    treatment 213-16
sinusitis 191-5
skin 12, 13, 16, 33, 34-5
    lymph nodes 94
    lymphatic malfunction 152, 172
    maintenance 196
smoking 101-2
snoring 25, 172, 183, 195
sore throat 4, 8, 20-1, 45
    antibiotics 48
    joint pain 177-8
    repair 24

self-help 47-8, 50
   tonsils 62, 64, 69, 70
spleen 5, 18, 22
sprains 224-5
squints 169-71
sterilization 43
steroids 110-11, 118, 197
sticky eye 162
stomach 67
streptococcal infections 151, 198
styes 162-3
subconscious 108-9
sugar 54-5, 122, 172
supplements 55-8, 111, 210, 224
sweating 34
swellings 24-6, 28, 198-200
swimming 32
sympathetic nerves 200-1

teeth 96, 138, 201-2
temperature 33-7
temporomandibular joint
   syndrome (TMJ) 201-3
temporomandibulitis 201-2
thoracic nodes 93, 98-100, 101-2
throat 13, 23-5, 33, 35-6
   antibiotics 50
   appendix 78-9
   cervical nodes 83, 84
   eczema 152-3
   self-help 39
   tonsils 61, 63
   treatment 218-19
thunderstorms 40
tinnitus 147-50
tissue fluid 11-13, 16, 20, 24-5, 27
tomatoes 172
tongue 35
tonsils 5, 9, 18, 19-21
   asthma 111, 114

cervical nodes 83
lymphatic structure 61-73
mental function 67-8
self-help 44, 47
toxins 203
trace elements 57-8, 181-2, 210
trachea 219
trampolines 32
travel sickness 204
treatment 27-9, 207-25
Turner, J M W 160

ulcers 204-6, 223-4
ultrasound 28, 47, 65, 95, 118
   treatment 212, 216, 218-19, 221,
      224-5
   waves 9, 139
use-by dates 43
uterus 95, 185, 221-2

vegetables 21, 43, 56, 64
vestibule 87
vestibulitis 151
viruses 5, 10, 12, 16
   antibiotics 46-7
   sterilization 43
   swollen membranes 25-6
vitamins 55-7, 64-5, 95, 114, 138, 210
vitreous humour 89-90
vulva 97, 221-2

weather 39-40
wheat 52-3, 172
white flour 172, 175
windpipe 219

yeast 172
yoghurt 51

zinc 58, 182